Pass the
MRCP
(Parts I and II)

All the techniques you need for the adult and paediatric exams

Mark Elliott

Donald Richardson

Keith Brownlee

Christopher Williams

W.B. Saunders Company Ltd
London Philadelphia Toronto Sydney Tokyo

W.B. Saunders Company Ltd
24–28 Oval Road
London NW1 7DX

The Curtis Center
Independence Square West
Philadelphia, PA 19106–3399, USA

Harcourt Brace & Company
55 Horner Avenue
Toronto, Ontario M8Z 4X6, Canada

Harcourt Brace & Company, Australia
30–52 Smidmore Street
Marrickville, NSW 2204, Australia

Harcourt Brace & Company, Japan
Ichibancho Central Building, 22–1 Ichibancho
Chiyoda-ku, Tokyo 102, Japan

A catalogue record for this book is available from the British Library

ISBN 0–7020–2198–9

Typeset by Keystroke, Jacaranda Lodge, Wolverhampton
Printed and bound in Great Britain by WBC Book Manufacturers, Bridgend,
Mid. Glamorgan

Contents

Contributors

Dr Mark Elliott   *Consultant in Respiratory Medicine, St James's University Hospital, Beckett Street, Leeds LS9 7TF, UK*

Dr Donald Richardson   *Registrar in Renal Medicine, St James's University Hospital, Beckett Street, Leeds LS9 7TF, UK*

Dr Keith Brownlee   *Consultant Paediatrician, St James's University Hospital, Beckett Street, Leeds LS9 7TF, UK*

Dr Chris Williams   *Lecturer/Honorary Senior Registrar in Psychiatry, St James's University Hospital, Beckett Street, Leeds LS9 7TF, UK*

The structure of this book is based on *Pass the MRCPsych* by Christopher Williams, Peter Trigwell and David Yeomans, published by W.B. Saunders. Several chapters and part chapters are reproduced from this with the permission of the authors.

Dr Peter Trigwell   *Senior Registrar in Psychiatry, Department of Liaison Psychiatry, Leeds General Infirmary, Leeds LS1 3EX, UK*

Dr David Yeomans   *Consultant Psychiatrist, Somerset House, Manor Lane, Shipley BD18 3BP, UK*

Dr Kevin Appleton   *Senior Registrar in Child and Adolescent Psychiatry, St James's Hospital, Beckett Street, Leeds LS9 7TF, UK*

Dr Siân McIver   *Registrar in Psychiatry, St James's Hospital, Beckett Street, Leeds LS9 7TF, UK*

Foreword
Professor Roy Meadow

Many books are available that contain past examination papers and illustrative questions. Most of them provide good ways of learning and revising, but few deal with the techniques and approaches that examinees collectively need to possess when they prepare for, and present themselves at, an examination. This book fills that gap, and provides various approaches that can be tailored to the needs of the individual candidate according to natural aptitudes and personal limitations.

The MRCP is the entry examination for specialist registrar training for Physicians and Paediatricians. Its aim is to ensure that those entering specialist training already have a certain level of knowledge and skill, without which they would not be able to make the most of their training. It provides a means of ensuring that trainees learn the basic facts, understand their scientific context, and amass the clinical experience that enables them to become competent specialists.

The book will be appreciated by candidates, and will be welcomed also by examiners. No examiner wishes a candidate to fail because of lack of exam technique or ignorance of understanding the rules. The MRCP is renowned for the scrupulous care which goes into its construction and the integrity with which it is conducted. However that thoroughness means that individual examiners have to award marks according to the strict rules of the exam and are not allowed to give the benefit of the doubt to a candidate who they think is underperforming because of lack of awareness of the way the exam is constructed or marked. Therefore this book, which clarifies the nature of the examination and which should help candidates to perform optimally, is to be welcomed.

Candidates who progress to the clinical stages of the Part II examination should remember that most of their examiners are committed and renowned teachers. Those examiners took the MRCP themselves years ago, and still remember the cases they encountered, the mistakes they made and the remarks made to them by their examiners. Because of that, most examiners try to use the examination as an opportunity to teach (compared with all the rest of their day-to-day teaching, they know that this is the one time when they have 100% of the trainees' attention, and that the information imparted will be remembered for ever). Therefore candidates should go into the exam prepared to learn. After each section of the exam look up the correct answers and discuss them with your colleagues. In the clinical exam, listen carefully to any words of wisdom from the examiner because you will remember that advice for the rest of your life. Moreover, there is nothing more discouraging for a committed teacher/examiner than a candidate who looks rather indignant, truculent or downcast, when one passes on a pearl of information or clinical advice that it has taken oneself several decades to learn. You are at the beginning of specialist training and are not expected to know everything. It is your job to show that you have the basic knowledge and skills with which to progress, *and* a willingness both to admit ignorance and to learn – which are qualities that every clinician needs throughout their career.

Professor Roy Meadows MA, BM, BCh, FRCP, DCH, DRCOG
Head of Department of Paediatrics and Child Health,
President of the British Paediatrics Association,
St James's University Hospital, Beckett Street,
Leeds, UK

Foreword
Professor Alex M Davison

The membership examination, both Part I and Part II, often seems to be an insurmountable hurdle for candidates. In part, this is because there is an aura surrounding the exam and many myths related about questions and examiners. In truth the exam does not set out with the intention of failing candidates, the examiners do not have some supernatural grasp of every nuance of clinical medicine and, in general, are no different from consultants of whom you will have experience, and the questions asked, in the main, deal with common clinical problems. This book provides much useful advice with respect to the examination and to the techniques of learning.

The development of the European Union has opened many opportunities for the medical profession and has also resulted in a reorganisation of postgraduate training. The examination for membership of the Royal Colleges of Physicians is unique and remains the best indicator of clinical knowledge and ability. Although the standard is high, with careful preparation the candidate should feel confident of success. This book will go a long way in helping those in the formative years of their career to achieve a pass thereby opening the road to their future.

Professor Alex M Davison BSc, MD, FRCP, Professor in Renal Medicine, St James's University Hospital, Beckett Street, Leeds, UK

Introduction

Clinical competence and passing the Membership examinations for the Royal Colleges of Physicians are the most visible criteria by which trainees progress up the career ladder in any branch of medicine or paediatrics. Taking the exams is costly in both financial and personal terms. To pass requires very significant work and commitment. The aim of this book is to provide a concise guide to all parts of the MRCP exam; it is the first book of its kind to focus on the important area of exam techniques.

This book is not a "crammer" book of key facts for the exam. You will find that very few factual pieces of information are presented. Instead, it will help you to present the information that you have learned elsewhere (whether from formal revision, everyday clinical practice or other sources) in a professional and structured way. Even very good clinicians with a strong factual knowledge may fail the exams because of poor technique. This book will help you to use your knowledge and experience effectively to enable you to pass. At the same time, we hope to help you develop the skills of a good clinician – someone who can manage their time, think quickly and efficiently, and present themselves professionally in exam and interview situations.

The book is divided into sections:

- Part I: Preparing for the exam

- Part II: The written exams

- Part III: The clinical exams

- Part IV: The Paediatric exam

We hope that you will find our book helpful. In producing any book such as this, many other people are always involved. In particular we would like to thank Professor Sandy Davison and Professor Roy Meadow, who have written the foreword to this book, and our colleagues who contribute to the MRCP teaching courses in Leeds.

Finally, but most importantly, we wish to thank Nicola, Alison, Catherine and Alison for their support and understanding during the writing of this book. Without this it would not have been possible.

Mark Elliott, Donald Richardson, Keith Brownlee,
Chris Williams

Part I

Preparing for the exam

Chapter 1

Important practical and preparation issues

Introduction

If you wish to pursue a career in some aspect of general internal medicine or paediatrics it will be necessary for you to sit, and pass, the exams that lead on to Membership of the Royal College of Physicians (MRCP). You will not get a place on a "Calman rotation" without Membership. Additionally, in many countries of the world, MRCP is highly regarded as a measure of clinical competence and in some countries, as in the UK, it is a hurdle that has to be successfully negotiated on the way to becoming a specialist. Before it is possible to sit either part of the Membership exam, there are specific requirements relating to how much time you have been in approved training in order for you to be eligible to sit the exam. You should obtain, and read, the examination regulations and information for candidates which are available from any of the Royal Colleges (for addresses see end of this chapter). You should read them particularly carefully if your career has been unusual in any way or if you are applying from abroad.

There are two parts to the exam.

- **Part I** is a multiple choice exam designed to assess quickly, reliably and fairly whether candidates have the basic knowledge necessary for the practice of medicine. It cannot be taken until 18 months after graduation, but it is probably best to take it as soon as you can, before too much of the basic science that you learnt as an undergraduate is forgotten. In addition, success will give you the edge in getting shortlisted for jobs.

- **Part II** is a more complex exam which further tests your knowledge, but additionally your reasoning ability, judgement, communication skills and clinical approach. It comprises a written paper, following which candidates who achieve a satisfactory standard will be invited to attend for the clinical exams.

Applying To Sit The Exams

You must request application forms from the College and submit these on time with the appropriate fee, payable in pounds sterling. The deadline is surprisingly early; you need to request the application forms several months in advance. It is not uncommon for candidates to "miss the boat" – book early to avoid disappointment and increased stress. For Part II, remember that you will need two testimonials at your first attempt, and one thereafter, either from Fellows or from Members of at least 8 years standing, of any of the Colleges.

Part I and the written section of Part II, can be sat in some countries other than the UK. Further details are obtainable from the Royal Colleges. The whole exam may be currently taken in Hong Kong, but only by doctors working there. Places are limited at all examination centres and it is therefore advisable to apply early.

Preparation

Once you have decided when to take the exam, immediately work out a **timetable** for revision. This can be detailed or simply a broad outline, depending on your preference. Try to mix subjects you find easy with more difficult areas and maintain variety. Be flexible – as you work through your revision if there are areas in which you are struggling, spend a bit more time on these and a bit less on those areas in which you are confident. **The timetable must be realistic and achievable**.

A timetable can inspire increased motivation to work, as you can see just what needs to be done and what areas need to be covered. It will also help to keep you on target for the exam if you stick to your timetable.

Most people assign a period of 3–6 months for revision for Part I and 6–9 months for Part II. It is helpful to work consistently, e.g. 2 hours a night, but be flexible to allow for relaxation, on-call commitments, and other occasions.

Many candidates find it helpful to decide upon a day each week when they will definitely not revise. Having regular breaks helps to maintain commitment the rest of the time. Remember to continue to have at least some social and "fun" activities. These will be a useful antidote to work.

It may help to structure your revision timetable by following one of the major textbooks. You will need a checklist of the subject areas to ensure that you cover everything required. It is useful steadily to build up a selection of stock answers for the clinical and oral exams.

Consider going on an examination course early in your revision. It can help you get a feel for what is required and may highlight from the outset potential weak areas which need particular work.

Do not burn yourself out and peak too early. Your preparations should be like that of an athlete getting ready for an important race. Increase the tempo as the exams approach, but keep something in reserve for the final weeks. Do not arrive at the exam feeling stale, jaded and having lost interest.

Benefits Of Addressing your Exam Techniques

Good preparation and adequate practice will enable you to feel confident that the exam is not going to bring too many surprises. It should also prevent you being thrown off balance by a difficult question, or at least enable you to function on "auto-pilot" until you regain your equilibrium. You should have pre-prepared answers and answering techniques for difficult questions. You should know how to impress examiners by your presentation technique. You should know the ins and outs of the exam structure and how it is marked. You should know what is expected of you. This will help to reduce your anxiety and improve your exam performance.

Practice

An analysis of your **learning style**, as described in Chapter 2, will shape the way you prepare for the exams. For every candidate without exception, however, **practice** is essential. It is important to test yourself regularly throughout the revision period in order to get feedback on your performance.

For Part I you will need to practise Multiple Choice Questions (MCQs). For the written section of Part II you will need to practise interpreting data and answering questions on case histories and on clinical material presented photographically. All these features should be built into your revision timetable.

For the clinical section of Part II you must practise **all** the parts of the exam. Candidates too often concentrate only on the short cases, both because these are perceived to be the most difficult part of the exam and because they lend themselves most easily to *ad hoc* teaching sessions.

Ask your peers and senior colleagues to listen to your presentations and give feedback. Be critical about their comments but do not take it all to heart. Each person you ask will have a slightly different opinion on what is good and bad about your efforts. Focus on what you find to be most helpful. With adequate practice you will have built up your confidence in your abilities before you enter the examination room.

Your Mental Health

Examinations cause stress over an extended period. It is worthwhile considering how the process is affecting you. Do you need a break? What about a holiday? Or a night out? What about relaxation, sport, television. If you do suffer from exam nerves it pays to practise relaxation beforehand. Do this in your mock exams too. Although some people have been known to find anxiolytics or beta-blockers helpful, medication should generally be avoided.

Last minute revision is sometimes more of an anxiolytic than an aid to memory. Do it if you have to, but a day of rest before the exams can also be therapeutic.

Practical Issues

- Make it easy on yourself. Get study leave arranged well in advance and stick to it. Consider attending a revision course. It may be helpful to take a week off work just before the exam for final preparations.

- Do not be persuaded to cover for an absent colleague at the last moment; you have spent too much time, effort and money to let personnel issues get in your way. Give yourself at least one clear day off work before travelling to the exam centre.

- If you are staying overnight, choose a comfortable hotel in a quiet location. It is worth the money. Do not skimp on last minute comforts, especially if you can claim expenses. Ring Personnel in advance to find out what you are entitled to. Some employers pay for revision courses too.

- Give yourself plenty of time to get to the exam centre. It is better to arrive 2 hours early than 2 minutes late. If you are late for any part of the exam it will leave you feeling tense, pressured and unlikely to perform well. It can destroy months of hard work, and mean that you will have to repeat all your revision once again.

- If using public transport, consider a back-up route if the service is disrupted. In general, if you start out early enough you can cope with traffic and rail delays. Consider flying longer distances. Pack in advance and do not rush.

- In the clinical exam, your personal presentation will earn marks. Dress appropriately. Be polite and courteous to everyone.

State of Mind on the Exam Day

To do well in the exams it helps not to be distracted. Some find it easy to concentrate, but others may need actively to focus on the exam and exclude thoughts of work, home and low confidence. Practise relaxation techniques if this helped during revision. Reassure yourself that all your preparation means you are at an advantage before the exam starts, and with luck you will have already prepared answers to some of the questions that will arise.

After the Exam

You will not know how things have gone, although you may feel elated or depressed at your performance. Certain parts of the exam leave the vast majority of candidates feeling that they have probably failed (although many obviously have not). These feelings may continue for some time. Try to avoid too many post-mortems. Going over your answers again and again in your mind, analysing possible mistakes, is rarely helpful. A holiday break away may be a good idea.

You have to wait a while for the results. If you pass, well done! If not, then **try again**, as many current Members and Fellows of the Royal Colleges have had to in the past. Take note of the feedback from the examiners and keep working on your exam technique. (See **Appendix 1: What if you fail? trying again**.)

Key points

- Obtain and read the exam regulations and information for candidates.

- Understand how they apply to you.

- When you have decided to take the exam, send off for the application forms early.

- Submit completed forms, with the appropriate fee, in good time.

- Formulate a comprehensive revision timetable, including time off for recreation, etc.

- Examination technique can help you communicate what you know to your best ability. Think carefully about this aspect of the exam.

- Practise, practise, practise.

Useful Addresses

Royal College of Physicians of Edinburgh
9 Queen Street, Edinburgh EH2 1JQ
Tel: 0131 225 7324

Royal College of Physicians and Surgeons of Glasgow
242 St Vincent Street, Glasgow G2 5RJ
Tel: 0141 221 6072

Royal College of Physicians of London
11 St Andrews Place, Regent's Park, London NW1 4LE
Tel: 0171 935 1174

Chapter 2

Learning styles and revision strategies

Introduction

It is often believed that success in medical examinations depends simply on the faithful regurgitation of facts. This is not the whole truth. It is certainly possible to know the facts of a subject very well and still fail the examination. You can significantly improve your exam performance, however, with good technique. Technique refers to your style of **learning** and **preparing**, and then of **using and presenting** the learnt information to best effect.

Membership examinations are complex and difficult. It may be some time since you have taken a major examination, or worked in the way required to prepare for such a challenge. During house jobs you may well have taken a break from formal study, choosing instead to develop your practical skills and learning about everyday clinical medicine. The first part of the Membership exam tests the breadth of your medical knowledge. You will need to focus on relearning the basic sciences again. This is an area you will probably have neglected since the days of your preclinical training. In view of this, it is particularly important to think specifically about learning styles and the way you will go about preparing to sit the exams. You must decide both what to learn and how to structure your learning, so that you are prepared for the examination.

Learning Styles and Revision Strategies

Sit back for a moment and consider **what you know about how you learn**. Do you think that you have a personal learning style? It is very likely that you do, since you have spent at least 20 years in education developing your own methods of study. For example, you probably found that your own lecture notes at university were very different from those of your friends.

The following is a list of questions about learning styles. Work through it point by point; it is designed to get you thinking about how you learn.

- Do you revise in a **suitable environment**? (For example, quiet, warm enough, well lit, minimum of disturbance.) How can you **improve** the environment?

- Do you **set goals**? (For example, learn the components of the cranial nerves today and test yourself tomorrow.)

- Do you **achieve these goals**?

- Do you **structure your learning**? There is no point revising material for the exam which is unlikely to be examined. More importantly, you must not miss out subjects that you will be expected to know about and understand.

- Do you know what **sources of information** you are most comfortable with? Some people use up-to-date textbooks and try to learn them very well; others prefer to use a mixture of smaller texts and journal articles. Do not forget to concentrate on the main areas; these are often overlooked as people become bogged down in the fine detail of more obscure topics.

- Can you **prioritise**? (For example, learn the common things before the esoteric.)

- Do you **keep the exam in mind while learning**? (to spot questions, rehearse stock answers and memorise information in the style appropriate to the exam).

- **How much information** can you take in at one go? (There is no point staring at a book when your concentration seems to have gone. Taking a break will help to consolidate what you have learned.)

- **How much repetition** do you need? (Does it help to read several accounts from differing books, perhaps followed by a re-read of your own notes to fix those facts in your memory? Alternatively, are you the type of person who prefers to learn just one or two books really well?)

- **Reinforcing your learning** can be helpful. Do you review areas you have already covered? Try to revise the topic again after one week and four weeks to check your understanding and memory.

- Do you **use your daily work to help you learn**? (For example, practising your clinical assessments, spending time reflecting on your differential diagnoses, and management plans. Do you write up case notes in exam format?)

- Are you **adequately motivated**? (Try to make this positive e.g. career progression or self-satisfaction, rather than negative, e.g. coercion, financial loss or fear and "failure avoidance".) Passing the exam requires commitment.

- **Do you compare yourself with others too much**? Many candidates seem to delight in upsetting the "opposition" during revision and exams, and it is important to have a personal sense of your own abilities (expect some degree of hysteria and gamesmanship on revision courses).

- Do you **review your progress**? Are you keeping to your revision timetable?

- Do you find it helpful to make your own detailed notes, or do you prefer to highlight important facts in your textbooks?

- Do you work best by yourself, or as part of a group? Consider meeting once weekly for several hours with other colleagues who are doing the exam. This can help you to practise parts of the exam (like MCQs) and clarify difficult areas, as well as offering a useful source of support.

Practice

- For every candidate, without exception, **practice** is essential.

- Familiarity with the **clinical** exam can be gained only through practice. Be merciless in your pursuit of exam practice. Take every opportunity you can to practise presenting cases (ward rounds, clinic, etc.). Ask senior colleagues to listen to your presentations and give feedback. Take what **you** find most useful from different approaches and remember that there is no single right way to present a case.

- These practice sessions should mirror the real exam situation as closely as possible, so that you will have built up your confidence in your abilities before you enter the examination room.

- Make sure that you do mock clinical exams on each of the **main areas** that are likely to arise in the exam; all specialties include a group of disorders that lend themselves well to exams and so come up time and time again.

- Seek supervised training in interviewing skills. If you can, watch yourself presenting on video. This is the most effective way of changing and has the added advantage that the actual exam will be no more stressful than this.

- It is important to test yourself regularly throughout the revision period in order to get feedback on your performance in the various different components of the **written** examinations. Such self-assessment should be built into your revision timetable.

- Use the copy of the assessment sheet used by the examiners in your clinical exam, and the advice the relevant College issues to examiners. (A consultant you know who is, or has been, an examiner may be able to help with this.)

- Practise presenting to **peers**, and also watch them presenting. Attempt to mark each other's performance with an assessment sheet. You will gain from seeing how others present their cases, and they will also learn from you.

- Seek mock exams with a variety of **different examiners** with different theoretical and clinical backgrounds. If there are any College examiners at the hospital where you work, it would be well worth arranging to carry out at least one exam with them as well. Be willing to accept their feedback and suggestions to change. Ultimately, however, you are seeking to develop a clinical interview and presentation style with which **you** are happy.

Presenting Information

Chapters 3–12 of this book address the best way to present yourself, and the information you will have learnt, in each individual section of the MRCP examinations. Much of the content of this book is based on our experience in these settings. The material has been used by many candidates, who have found it helpful for their examinations. We hope that you find this too.

Key points

- Passing the exam requires a clear revision strategy.

- Exam techniques can be vital.

- Think about the way you learn: is it as effective as it could be?

- Revise with the exam in mind.

- Use your daily work to help you learn.

- Practice is essential.

Part II

The written exams

Chapter 3

The MRCP Part I multiple choice question exam

Introduction

Trainee doctors can fail the MRCP exam as a result of poor multiple choice question (MCQ) technique. It is possible for any candidate sitting a negatively marked exam to know the subject well, answer 72% of the questions correctly, and yet obtain a mark of only 44%. As a result, even some very knowledgeable clinicians fail the exam.

The MCQ paper is the most structured of all the exams, and aims to test the candidate's factual knowledge quickly and reliably. It is ironic that the negatively marked MCQ is probably more dependent on exam technique than most other forms of assessment. It is necessary to have a suitable depth of knowledge of the subjects in order to pass. This chapter suggests ways of planning your learning with the MCQ exam in mind, and also describes methods to improve your MCQ technique so that you are able to use your knowledge more effectively.

The MRCP Part I exam may be taken in either General Medicine or Paediatrics. The exam consists of 60 MCQs, 30 of which are the same for the General Medicine and the Paediatrics exam. There is no substitute for a thorough understanding of the subject matter.

There is no set pass mark, and 30% of candidates are allowed to pass at each sitting. Therefore if you fail this does not mean you have performed poorly.

Preparing For the Exam

- Produce a clear revision timetable in order to cover each area adequately. You will need to start your revision **well before** the exam if you are going to cover all the subject areas.

- It is often useful to go on a **Part I course** at the very beginning of your revision. There are several advantages. It can help you get your revision going, boost your motivation and highlight areas of weakness on which to focus your learning. It allows you to realise the depth of knowledge that you must aim for and the amount of time you need to set aside for your revision.

There is currently no examination syllabus, although one is being written by the Royal College of Physicians. When it is published, obtain and read it. It will state the areas the College (and hence the examiners) believes are important.

The following topics have repeatedly been included in both exams:

- Elementary statistics.
- Epidemiology.
- Clinical sciences.
- Basic sciences.

Subjects can include:

- Relevant principles of cell biology.

- Molecular biology.

- Membrane biology.

- Immunology.

- Genetics.

- Biochemistry.

- Anatomy.

- Physiology.

- Microbiology.

- Pharmacology.

Exclusive Paediatrics topics can include:

- Embryology.

- Fetal and child physiology.

- Child and adolescent growth.

- Child development.

- Child and family psychology.

Clearly it would be **impossible** to obtain an individual textbook on each of these subjects and to read it to the depth necessary to answer every MCQ. The best way of approaching this problem is therefore to choose a relatively simple system-specific text-book. Read it from cover to cover, trying to understand the **basic principles** thoroughly. Textbooks that cover the core subjects well include:

General Medicine:

- Davidson's Principles and Practice of Medicine[1]

- Lecture notes in Medicine[2]

- Souhami and Moxham[3]

- The Medicine Series[4]
- Kumar and Clark[5]

Paediatrics:

- Lecture notes in Paediatrics[6]
- Essential Paediatrics[7]
- Hospital Paediatrics[8]

This list is not exhaustive, but indicates the sort of level of knowledge that you should be seeking to acquire. You will need to **supplement** this reading with other more focused learning from a variety of other sources. These should include more specialised textbooks and basic science textbooks.

You must make sure that you feel comfortable with the style and "readability" of your main book as it is likely that you will end up reading large parts of it several times.

How To Use MCQs To Help You Revise

At the beginning of your preparation for the exam it useful to spend some time **writing** MCQs. For example, after completing a chapter of a book, try to write a few MCQs on the subject you have just learned. This helps to **reinforce** and test your knowledge and will help **highlight** the kind of information that is amenable to MCQs. The questions are also useful for later revision.

As you read through your textbooks, mark facts which are MCQ-able with a **highlighter pen**. The number of black and white or true–false facts are remarkably limited. This will help you focus your learning.

Remember that the information needed to answer MCQs is quite different from that needed to "manage a patient".

A large variety of MCQ books are available. Some of these are better (and more accurate) than others. Some books contain whole papers of mixed questions; others consist of questions organised by topic. Both of these formats are very helpful, but should be used in different ways. The most useful MCQs are those published by the College.[9]

- Make sure that you attempt some MCQs published by the College **at the start of your revision**. This will set a standard to revise to.

- **Make your revision more interesting** by using MCQs. Some people find that when they continually revise a set of notes over a period of weeks they cease to take in any new information. One way of preventing this is to practise MCQs on each topic shortly after you have revised it.

- Remember that MCQs are a very valuable source of MCQ-able information. **Improve your factual knowledge base** by reading and testing yourself with as many MCQs as you can. If you find you do badly in a particular subject or topic, target your reading towards these areas. You can then re-read the topic, looking for the answers to the questions that you got wrong. This helps highlight particular areas of a subject as important, and allows you to add important details to your notes.

- Do not try to remember hundreds of dislocated facts. Instead try to **integrate** information you learn with your existing knowledge so that you **understand** the **principles** involved. **Summary notes** may help you do this. Of most value are books that **explain** the answers, so that you add to your knowledge.

Subject Spotting

Exam courses often make a lot of subject spotting. By analysing previous papers and reporting the apparent frequency of different subjects, it is suggested that it is possible to target revision at specific exam-oriented subjects. This is generally of limited value as the content of different exams varies significantly. It is clear, however, that there are certain core subject areas that you must know and understand well.

Core Subject Areas

(Most Medicine and Paediatrics textbooks cover these clinical subjects well.)

- Cardiology.
- Haematology.
- Respiratory system.
- Neurology.
- Endocrinology.
- Gastroenterology.
- Nephrology.
- Pharmacology.
- Infectious diseases.
- Immunology.
- Psychiatry.
- Rheumatology.
- Oncology.
- Growth and development (Paediatrics only).
- Neonatology (Paediatrics only).

While you must have a good knowledge of the core subjects, most candidates concentrate on these and pay inadequate attention to the less common topics. Building these into your study plan could give you an advantage. Time spent on the fringe subjects may be very productive. The College database has fewer questions on these topics, they tend to be more straightforward, and are often present in the MCQ books.

"Fringe" subjects include:

- Ophthalmology.

- Nutrition.

- Surgery.

- Tropical medicine.

- Sports medicine.

- Statistics.

- Molecular biology.

- Cell biology.

- Genetics.

- Embryology (Paediatrics only).

Most readable Medicine and Paediatrics textbooks do not cover these subjects in sufficient detail to allow you to answer very specific MCQs. You must therefore **supplement your reading with more specialised texts** in these areas.

It is well worth paying disproportionate attention to particular conditions, questions about which appear **more frequently** in MCQ exams than they do in clinical practice. These include topics such as:

- Tuberculosis and tuberculin testing.

- Acquired immune deficiency syndrome.

- Systemic lupus erythematosus.

- Salmonella.

- Brucellosis.

- Sarcoidosis.

- Hodgkin's disease.

- Fibrosing alveolitis.

- Renal tubular acidosis.

- Porphyrias.

- Malaria and tropical medicine.

- Glucose-6-phosphate dehydrogenase deficiency.

- Sickle cell disease.

- Thalassaemia.

- Cushing's syndrome.

- Lung cancer.

- Bronchopulmonary aspergillosis.

If there is only 1 hour left to study before the exam, it would be more productive to read several of these topics in detail than skip through a very large area such as cardiology.

Testing Your "Feeling of Knowing"

In the MCQ exam, one mark will be awarded for each correct answer, zero marks for a "don't know" response, and minus one for an incorrect response. This negative marking approach was introduced to discourage candidates from guessing. In theory, if you haven't a clue about the answer, a complete guess should have an equal chance of being correct or incorrect, thus resulting in an average of zero marks. In practice, however, **some people seem to be**

naturally better at answering MCQs than others and will score highly because of their ability to make a confident calculated guess. One area that has been researched is the "**feeling of knowing**" that candidates experience when they read certain questions. When you do an MCQ paper, you will find that you either:

- **Know** the answer with a high degree of certainty.

- Definitely know that you **don't know** the answer.

- Have a "**feeling of knowing**" that the answer is correct, but are **not quite sure**.

Studies show that the accuracy of people's "feeling of knowing" varies. Even allowing for negative marking, most people will finish up with a net positive mark if they act in response to their "gut" feelings concerning the "right" answer. **It is important to know whether this general statistical finding is true for you**. It is our experience that approximately one in eight candidates are not able to trust their "feeling of knowing". For whatever reason, if they trust their "gut" feeling, they will be more often wrong than right. **This can have disastrous results in the exam**. If you have found that throughout your exam career you have persistently experienced problems passing negatively marked MCQs, you may be one of these people. You need to find out whether you are, because this has important implications for how you should approach the exam.

To find this out, do several MCQ papers covering a range of topics. As you do each paper, mark your answers using either a black or a red pen:

- If you know the answer, mark it in **black**.

- If you don't know the answer, leave it **blank**.

- If you have a "feeling of knowing" mark it in **red**.

Now go through the papers and mark them in order to compare your mark when you were certain, and what additional score you would obtain when you use your "feeling of knowing". Try this on a number of papers. If you find that, on average, you have a net gain of marks by using your instincts, keep doing it. If not, then be cautious about answering questions on a negatively marked paper unless you are at least reasonably sure about the answer.

- If your "certain" answers are wrong, you may be **overconfident** about your knowledge and need to do more factual revision.

- If you have problems with MCQ papers, you will need to **repeat this process on a large number of papers** to try to identify what strategy is the most effective for you. Repeated practice will help you to be confident of your answering technique.

The MCQ Exam

Timing and practical issues

Check the up-to-date College examination instructions and regulations to find out how many questions you have to complete and what time is allocated. The structure and content of the exam may change. Currently, 2.5 hours are allowed for the exam. This is more than enough to complete the paper. You are expected to complete 60 MCQs made up of five stems per question (300 stems in total), and should aim to complete 10 questions approximately every 20 minutes. This will allow you 30 minutes at the end to check your answers.

MCQ technique

- **Read the whole question very carefully** and break it down into individual facts. Mark each of these facts as true or false. Read each stem and item as a single sentence.

- Be particularly careful with questions on topics about which you are confident. Your elation may lead you to misread the question and lose marks where you should have gained them. A colleague in Finals had made a particular point of learning the anatomical relations of the ureter. He was delighted, therefore, to find this exact question. Unfortunately he gained no marks because the question was about the anatomical relations of the urethra.

- Have you understood the question? Beware of double negatives – one in the question and one in the stem.

- Make sure you put each answer straight away on to the right line of the answer sheet. Check this every question. It is easy to get your answers out of order. This will cause panic and could cost you the exam. Avoid it.

- **Ruthlessly skip questions where you really don't know the answer** and come back to them later. It is likely that you will find other questions easier. Answer what you can, and then carry on. You may find that other questions trigger your memory, and the answer will come back to you as the exam continues.

- **Review your progress regularly** to make sure that you complete the paper.

There is a move towards producing questions that present information in the stem as a clinical scenario. In essence these are no different from conventional questions.

Example

A 15-year-old boy presents with a sudden onset of wheezing, shortness of breath and cough. He has had no previous respiratory *symptoms. His heart rate is 110 per minute and the respiratory rate is 40. Auscultation of his chest revealed coarse wheeze and his peak flow was 400 l/min. Arterial blood gas analysis shows a Pa CO_2 of 3.4 kPa, Pa O_2 of 12.8 kPa in air and pH 7.48.*

(a)   He is having an acute severe episode of asthma.
(b)   He requires oxygen urgently.
(c)   He should be given intravenous aminophylline.
(d)   He requires an urgent chest radiograph.
(e)   Pulsus paradoxus would be a valuable measure in this child.

There is a lot of information in this question which needs to be considered.

- Is he having an asthma attack?

- Is it an acute severe asthma attack?

- Does he require oxygen?

- Does he require oxygen urgently?, etc.

By approaching each part of the question logically, a good attempt can be made at the question.

Don't be too clever

Do not automatically assume that the examiners are trying to trick you. **Avoid agonising over possible hidden meanings**, as this is more likely to hinder rather than help your decisions.

In MCQs, the "correct" answer to a question is the **generally accepted version of the truth**. If you have some special knowledge of a topic which is at variance with the most prevalent viewpoint, swallow your pride and save it for the viva.

Example

The following facts about our solar system are true:

(a)   It takes 365 days for the Earth to orbit the Sun.

(b) The same side of the Moon is always visible from the Earth.
(c) The moon circles the Earth every 28 days.
(d) Gravity is related to the speed of rotation of a planet.
(e) Only planets with an iron core have a magnetic field.

- The answer to stem **(a)** is true; however, the very knowledgeable candidate may be aware that the Earth takes 365.27 days to circulate the Sun, he or she may then answer this as false.

- The same side of the moon is always visible from Earth, therefore stem **(b)** is true; however, there is a phenomenon called libration as a consequence of which 59% of the Moon's surface is visible, but at different times. If the candidate is aware of this, he or she may then answer this question incorrectly as false. This is reading to much into the question.

- The answer to stem **(c)** is true. However, the very knowledgeable candidate may be aware that the Moon takes 27.3 days to circulate the Earth; he or she may then answer this as false. This is being too precise.

- The answer to stem **(d)** is false. Gravity is related to the mass of an object. This is a question you can answer only if you have specific knowledge about this fact.

- **Dichotomous statements** such as "**only**" and "**always**" and "**never**" often indicate that the answer is false. It is very rare for a finding to occur absolutely only in one situation. The answer to stem **(e)** is therefore likely to be (and in fact is) false.

It is also possible to be too clever by adding to the information that you have been given. With a little bit of ingenuity and lateral thinking it is possible to make almost anything true!

Example

Cough is a recognised feature of hypertension.
The answer is "false". However, you could argue that angiotensin converting enzyme (ACE) inhibitors are often used to treat hypertension and may cause cough, and therefore that cough is a recognised feature of hypertension. Avoid adding conditions, however reasonable they may seem. **Answer the question as it is written**.

The numbers game

- There is no set pass mark. A candidate's performance is compared with all other candidates taking the exam on that occasion. In practice, the pass mark is usually between 55 and 60%. This will require you to score at least 160 correct items (out of 300).

- Don't decide beforehand how many questions you are going to answer. **Answer as many as you can**; however, if you answered a lot below 200 questions, you may have to make a few more calculated guesses.

- If you are finding the paper horrendously difficult, it is likely that others are too. **Do not give up**. Carry on and try to finish. Do not leave the exam hall in despair. You can still pass.

Be Aware of the Techniques Examiners Use in Writing Questions

It is surprisingly difficult to write good MCQs. Understanding some of the techniques used will help you to avoid some of the possible pitfalls. It is useful to think about questions from the perspective of the person writing them. They will wish to have a spread of true and false responses, of varying degrees of difficulty. Ideally the questions will be able to discriminate between those who know a subject well and those whose knowledge is superficial. Unfortunately for you the techniques used to construct questions may mean that a little knowledge can make it more likely that the incorrect answer is chosen – this is particularly true when the correct answer is "false".

It is **relatively easy to formulate "true" questions**. Read a chapter in a textbook and see how easy it is to pick out five facts that are true. The question can be made more difficult either by choosing obscure facts or by expressing the question in a form that is unlikely to have been read in a textbook, but can be worked out if the subject is known well. It is possible that you will sometimes know the answer to a question but not realise it. This is because the question has been **phrased in an unexpected way** or because it occurs in an unexpected place.

Example

In a patient with pulmonary oedema due to cardiomyopathy:

(a) The hydrogen ion concentration may be raised.

In your reading about cardiac disease you will probably **not** have read about the effects of a low cardiac output on acid–base homoeostasis. However, in reading about metabolic abnormalities **you will have read** that poor perfusion is associated with lactic acidosis. In addition, you are probably much more familiar with dealing with pH and will have read about the effect of poor perfusion on pH. You ought to be able to work out that a high hydrogen ion concentration is the same as a low pH. You should therefore be able to work out that the answer is "true", even if you initially thought that you did not know the answer.

Overall, you should be confident about your "true" answers; after all you are answering it as "true" because you have seen or heard it somewhere before. **It is much more difficult to be confident about your "false" answers**. The fact that you think that "A is not a feature of B" may simply reflect that you do not know much about the subject.

Example

Multiple sclerosis is more common in owners of "lap" dogs than in those of Great Danes.

It should be possible to answer this confidently as "false" because you have never seen it written in any textbook as being an important factor in the aetiology of multiple sclerosis and it sounds fairly outrageous. Unfortunately it is true and used to be cited as evidence that multiple sclerosis was caused by a transmissible agent from dogs.

It is much more difficult for the examiners to write good "false" questions. They may be created by using **popular misconceptions** or by using the **opposite** of the truth. **Candidates are more likely not to answer a question if the correct answer is "false"** rather than if it is "true". Therefore, being able to answer the "false" questions correctly can give you the edge over other candidates and be a very valuable source of extra marks. To answer a question as "false" requires an extensive knowledge of the subject and you need to be more careful when answering "false" than "true", except when you recognise that a "switch" has occurred and you know that the opposite is true.

Recognising the switch

The following can be switched:

1. Nouns (or diseases).

2. Adjectives.

3. Negative to positive, or vice versa.

Example

The following statements are true about the planets:

(a)   Jupiter has a great dark spot.
(b)   The hottest planet is Mercury.

The answer to stem **(a)** is false. If the candidate remembers that Jupiter has a spot, he or she may well answer this as true; unfortunately, Jupiter has a red spot, Neptune has a dark spot. This stem has been created by **switching words** or by **mixing known facts**. Here, a little knowledge is likely to make an "educated" guess wrong.

The answer to stem **(b)** is false. If the candidate knows that Mercury is the nearest planet to the sun, he or she may answer this question as true. Venus, the second nearest planet to the sun, is, however, the hottest because it possesses an atmosphere and is affected by the greenhouse effect. This question has been created by **switching key words**.

Example

The following statements are true about atypical pneumonia:

(a) *Legionella* can be caught from parrots.
(b) Psittacosis pneumonia is associated with haemolytic anaemia.
(c) Mycoplasma pneumonia is associated with lung abscesses.
(d) Cold agglutinins are typical of *Legionella*.
(e) *Mycoplasma* is associated with a "rose spot rash".

If the candidate knows that:

- It is possible to contract atypical pneumonia from birds (psittacosis).

- Haemolytic anaemia and cold agglutinins occur in one of the atypical pneumonias (*Mycoplasma*).

- Lung abscesses are a complication of unusual pneumonias (*Klebsiella*).

- A rose spot rash occurs in some infections (*Chlamydia*).

it is possible that he or she may make a calculated guess that the above statements are true. In fact they are all false. The questions have been constructed by taking a known fact and **exchanging a**

key word. It is important that candidates are aware of this technique for writing questions and the pitfalls it may cause.

Example

In excessive antidiuretic hormone secretion:

(a)   Plasma osmolarity is increased.
(b)   Urinary sodium concentration is low.
(c)   Ankle oedema is likely to occur.
(d)   Head injury is not a cause.
(e)   Is unlikely to follow major surgery.

All of these answers are false. The question has been created by reading a textbook, picking out facts and "**switching**" the correct answer. If they are recognised as a switch, the statement can be answered as false.

Example

Wolf–Parkinson–White (WPW) syndrome is associated with a long PR interval.

You know, or should do, that WPW syndrome is associated with a **short** PR interval. It is therefore easy to recognise that the opposite is true and that this answer is therefore false.

The Wording of the Question

It is important to look at questions from two perspectives: factual knowledge and logic. If the questions are well written then it should be impossible to answer them without any knowledge of the subject. However, good MCQs are difficult to write and many questions contain some clues within the structure of the question. Use your common sense.

Three particularly common stems are:

- A "**characteristic feature**" means that it is of diagnostic significance. Its absence might make one doubt the diagnosis. If it is truly characteristic then you are likely to be aware of it.

- A **"typical feature"** is one which you would expect to be present. It is similar to "characteristic".

- A **"recognised feature"** is one that, although it may not characterise a disease, has been reported. For this to be false implies an in-depth knowledge of the subject, unless it can be recognised as a switch.

Other terminology

- **"Is a pathognomonic feature"** means it occurs only in that condition. If you do not know the answer then it is likely to be false. There are few pathognomonic features and you are likely to know them.

- **"Is associated with"** means that it is a feature that is well recognised but not common. The same applies to as a **"recognised feature of"**.

- Categorical answers such as **"never, always, only, invariably"** should be answered as false, unless you are sure that they are true.

Confusing and often ambiguous terminology

- **"Probably, frequent, often, likely"**, etc. – these tend to be false.

- **"Possible, may, rarely, can"**, etc. – these tend to be true.

Use your sense of logic

The following techniques may help you clarify your thinking about an answer:

1. Look for terminology that is likely to make a question true or false.
2. Look for **contradictions** between items.
3. Beware of double negatives.
4. Reversing the question (e.g. "X **may not** occur in Y") can help clarify your thinking. Try this with some questions in any MCQ book to illustrate how helpful this technique is.

Example

In phaeochromocytoma:

(a) There is unlikely to be a family history of the disease.

Reversing the question leads to "*In phaeochromocytoma there may be a family history*". This will make it more likely that you would answer "true" correctly.

5. Look for items that are **contradictory** or the same. Contradictory items should not be included within one question as they will be immediately obvious. However, they may be included in different questions, and this can offer you additional clues.

Example

In ketoacidosis:

(a) The pH is likely to be low.	(True)
(b) The hydrogen ion concentration is likely to be low.	(False)
(c) There is a decrease in organic acids.	(False)

Clearly all of these items cannot be true.

- The answer to (a) and (b) **cannot** be the same.

- The answer to (a) and (c) is **unlikely** to be the same.

Summary

Using these techniques may help you gain some further marks, but there is no substitute for developing a broad based knowledge.

Key points

- Make sure you know the structure of the exam.

- Start your revision early.

- Read lots of MCQs and commit yourself on paper.

- Practise using a variety of MCQ books and use MCQs to help you revise.

- Initially concentrate on a solid understanding of the subject matter.

- Work to perfect your technique.

- Read the questions very carefully.

- Test whether you can trust your "feeling of knowing".

- Don't panic: exam papers often seem very hard.

- Read the questions carefully, looking for clues in the wording.

- Keep checking your answers are in the correct place on the answer sheet.

- Maintain momentum.

References

[1] J. Macleod, C. Edwards and L. Bouchier (Ed.), *Davidson's Principles and Practice of Medicine*, 17th edn, Churchill Livingstone, London, 1995.

[2] H. Rubenstein and D. Wayne, *Lecture notes on Clinical Medicine*, Blackwell, Oxford, 1994.

[3] R. L. Souhami and J. Moxham, *Textbook of Medicine*, Churchill Livingstone, London, 1994.

[4] Medicine International (published yearly), The Medicine Group (UK) Ltd. 62 Stert Street, Abingdon, Oxon OX14 3UQ.

[5] P. Kumar and M. Clark, *Clinical Medicine*, 3rd edn, Bailliere Tindall, London, 1994.

[6] S. R. Meadows and R. W. Smithells, *Lecturing notes in Paediatrics*, 6th edn, Blackwell Science, London, 1993.

[7] D. Hull and D. I. Johnstone, *Essential Paediatrics*, Churchill Livingstone, London, 1993.

[8] A. D. Milner and D. Hull, *Hospital Paediatrics*, 2nd edn, Churchill Livingstone, London, 1992.

[9] MRCP (UK) Part I Examining Board, *MRCP (UK). Part I Papers. Multiple Choice Question Papers from the MRCP (UK) Part I examination.* Royal College of Physicians of Edinburgh, Royal College of Physicians and Surgeons of Glasgow, Royal College of Physicians of London, Margate, 1991.

Chapter 4

The MRCP Part II written exams

Introduction

The written section of the MRCP Part II exam consists of three papers with equal marks assigned to each part. It is not necessary to achieve a particular mark for each as long as the aggregate for all three reaches the required level. It is possible to proceed to the clinical exams with a marginal fail in the writtens. In this case, you will have to make up these marks in the clinical in order to pass overall. A thorough factual knowledge of medicine is necessary but not sufficient. **Technique is essential** in order to do well in the written paper, as in every other part of the MRCP exam.

The three papers are:

1. **Case histories** (time allowed 55 minutes) – four or more case histories are presented with the results of physical examination and investigations. Physical signs, radiology and pathology may also be presented as photographs, or described. The questions are designed to test your diagnostic skills and your ability to plan further appropriate investigations and outline a management plan.

2. **Data interpretation** (time allowed 45 minutes) – ten questions consisting of laboratory or graphical

data. This tests not only your understanding of a range of biochemical and physiological processes, but also how well you are able to integrate information and to summarise your answers clearly and concisely.

3. **Photographic material** (time allowed 50 minutes) – 20 questions each based upon printed photographs of patients, radiographs and occasionally pathological specimens.

Revising for the Written Exams

During your revision you should be developing:

- Knowledge.

- Judgement.

- Precision in answering questions.

As with the first part of the Membership exams, there is no substitute for **knowledge**. There is no syllabus as such at present, and consequently it can be difficult to decide exactly what to learn. You may be presented with:

- Rare disorders.

- Unusual manifestations of common conditions.

- Cases from everyday practice.

Ideally you should have a very detailed knowledge of one of the large general medical textbooks (e.g. The Oxford Textbook of Medicine[1]), supplemented by detailed further reading in large specialist books. **Do not despair**. This is clearly not possible. It is a popular misconception that you need to know all about everything. You should aim instead to have a **working knowledge** across all the General Medical or Paediatrics specialities as a basic foundation of knowledge, and should supplement this with more detailed study in specific areas.

- Read one of the undergraduate medical textbooks for adult medicine and paediatrics from cover to cover (e.g. *Davidson's Principles and Practice of Medicine*[2], Kumar and Clarke[3], Souhami and Moxham[4], *Lecture notes on Clinical Medicine*[5], *Lecture notes in Paediatrics*[6] or *Hospital Paediatrics*[7]). You will find it relatively easy and it will give you a broad knowledge base. The Medicine series[8] is also useful and has the advantage of being regularly updated.

- Spread your learning effectively. Your more detailed study should span as many specialties as possible. Remember that it is an exam that tests your General Medical knowledge. You should avoid getting bogged down trying to learn one or two subjects in very great detail and neglecting completely other areas of medicine. While you might wish to become a great authority on the minutiae of, for instance, cardiology, this will not help you with most of the questions. **Broadly speaking you should cover the same specialties as were recommended for Part I of the exam**.

- It is useful to read the **clinicopathological cases** in the *New England Journal of Medicine* or the occasional similar cases such as the "Lesson of the Week" and the "Grand Rounds" in the *British Medical Journal*. From these you can learn from experts how to weigh and judge information and come to a diagnosis. In addition, it is an interesting way to learn about unusual cases.

- The papers contain a number of questions common to both Paediatrics and General

Medicine, enabling the examiners to compare the performance of both categories of candidates. This ensures that there is no variation in standard between the General Medicine and Paediatrics papers. It is therefore important that you do not confine your revision exclusively to the paper that you are sitting. The questions found in both exams will be relevant to practice within both specialties, dealing with problems that are likely to be found at the interface between paediatric and adult medical practice or illnesses in which the presentation is similar in both.

Example

Conditions that occur in adolescence (cystic fibrosis, diabetes, asthma, tuberculosis, etc.).

Use of exam practice books

One way of maintaining variety, and keeping your study broadly based, is to use the large number of books of questions, data interpretation and photographic material aimed at candidates sitting for the MRCP exam. Several of these books are unfortunately poorly written and contain factual mistakes.

- These have the advantage that they will familiarise you with some of the rare conditions you may come across in the exam and are a welcome diversion from struggling through textbooks.

- Exam-oriented books can be used to **stimulate more detailed reading** in larger general or specialist textbooks, and also help you to **focus** your learning on areas that are common in the exam.

- It is a mistake to rely exclusively on these specialist Membership books or on books of lists. You will have a greater chance of getting the right answer by **understanding** subjects rather than learning facts by rote.

- The **books of past papers** compiled and edited by the MRCP (UK) Part II Examining Board[9], published in 1986 and 1994, are **mandatory reading**. These will show you the standard that is required and it is very important that, having answered the questions, you carefully read the specimen answers. This will help you to understand the high degree of precision that is required in answering the questions.

- One useful approach is to obtain both sets of papers, using one at the beginning and retaining the other to use as a mock exam towards the end of your revision. You will still need to use other books of "Membership" pictures, cases, data interpretation, etc., mentioned above, but remember that some books are much easier and some much harder than the actual exam. Starting with one of the past papers published by the Royal College of Physicians will help you to set your performance in these other books against the necessary standard and to **structure your revision to the level that is required**.

The Membership exam is not just about learning facts, but also about how you **use your knowledge effectively** as a good clinician. Many candidates expect the written exam to be a straightforward regurgitation of factual knowledge in the form of a list. They are surprised how difficult it is to complete the questions fully, even when the question is about a topic with which that particular candidate feels very familiar. As in clinical practice there may be a number of correct answers, but you may be asked for only one. In other words your **judgement** will also be tested. It is therefore important that you develop the skill of selecting the most likely from a list of possibilities. For instance, you may know a long list of causes of hepatosplenomegaly, but not be able to select the one that most closely fits the information you have been given.

The examiner does not make a decision as to whether each of the questions is passed or failed. You can get the diagnosis wrong but still get the investigations right. **You can pick up marks from any and all parts of each question**; these are then simply added up to decide whether or not you pass the paper overall.

You may have excellent knowledge and develop a good sense of judging between the correct and the more correct and yet still fail the written part of the exam, because of a failure to understand how the exam is marked. Marks are awarded in a predetermined manner and very specific answers are required. Correct answers will receive maximum marks, but vague, incomplete or partly wrong answers will score lower or no marks. It is possible to know the correct answer, but fail to get the maximum number of available marks because you were **not sufficiently precise**. For instance, if given some arterial blood gases to interpret, "metabolic acidosis" would score more marks than "acidosis", etc. If shown a photograph of a radiograph and the correct answer is "left pneumothorax" the candidate will probably only get half marks (or at least lose some marks) if he or she only writes down "pneumothorax".

The Exam Itself

1. General points to consider

- It is essential to arrive in plenty of time for the paper.

- Legibility is essential. Each examiner will be marking many Part II papers. They will not be happy with any paper which includes illegible answers needing to be deciphered. The possible result is a very low mark which does not reflect the candidate's true level of knowledge, nor the amount of effort they have put in when preparing for the exam.

- Some **abbreviations** are so universally used that they are acceptable answers. ECG, CXR are possible examples of this type but **if in any doubt at all it is worth writing out all of the answer in long-hand**. Other, less universal, abbreviations are not safe to use. For example, TOF is commonly used, but could be taken to mean tracheo-oesophageal fistula (TOF) or tetralogy of Fallot (TOF).

- Before starting each section of the exam carefully **read the instructions** and listen to any comments made by the invigilators.

- Check that your examination number is printed at the top right-hand corner of each answer page of the question book and note that you are not allowed to remove question papers from the examination room.

- The question papers must **not be copied**, nor can you make notes on scrap paper. You are, however, allowed to write anywhere on the question book.

- All the questions must be answered.

2. Time awareness

- Make sure you know the time that has been allocated for each section of the exam and how many questions have to be answered. Calculate the amount of time you have per question, and stick to this rigidly.

- Make a prompt start. If the first one or two questions appear particularly tricky, you should **move on** to later questions and come back to the first ones later.

- Read the complete question before answering any part.

- You must be **constantly aware** of the time. Make a point of stopping after approximately half the questions are completed to see how the time is going.

- If certain questions seem easy for you **do not spend too long** on them. There may be a temptation to put in too much information. A straightforward answer will probably get you the marks; you should press on as you will find the extra time valuable when grappling with the more difficult questions. **However, make sure you have not missed the point**.

- Allow yourself some time to review your answers at the end of the paper.

3. Calm approach

A few of the questions will seem especially difficult. You may find that you are not sure what the question is asking for and so do not feel able to proceed with **any** of that question. **Do not panic**. Move on and return to that question later. Try to allow time to do so, as the answer may suddenly become clearer later on. Remember that any question which seems very hard for you is probably very hard for everyone.

4. Think yourself into the situation

Try to imagine you are encountering this problem in everyday clinical practice in Casualty or Outpatients. Decide what you would do in clinical practice. Try to forget that you are in an exam.

5. Broad or divergent thinking

Another reason why candidates grind to a premature halt is the use of **narrow thinking**. Any particular question is likely to produce a few instant and, to the candidate, obvious answers. After writing them down, however, there may not appear to be any other answers and full marks will not be gained. It is very important to forget the view *"that's all I seem to be able to think of"* and instead take the view *"if they're asking for six points then I know six points"*. The way to get access to the remaining answers is to make a conscious effort to **broaden your thinking**.

The way to broaden your thinking is to **consider what area of your knowledge you are actually using to answer the question**. You may be able to add to your answer by **switching to other areas**. Consciously **broadening** your approach to include other **subspecialty** areas can help. For example, you may be approaching it from the point of view of respiratory medicine, when a switch to thinking from the point of view of medicine for the elderly would stimulate further answers – for further marks.

A similar technique is to think of the headings of the "**surgical sieve**" in order to stimulate more answers. This is particularly useful in questions about **aetiology**. Typical headings used in this approach are:

- Inherited.
- Congenital.
- Metabolic.
- Infective.
- Inflammatory.
- Vascular.
- Neoplastic.
- Toxin or drug.
- Degenerative.

- Traumatic.

- Nutritional.

It may be that a return to first principles would help when at first the question seems obscure.

6. Take note of the number of responses requested

The examination has been designed to minimise the amount of writing and it is of no use to treat the questions as short essays in which you attempt to explain your thoughts to the examiner.

- If the question asks for two diagnoses, there will be two lines (one for each answer) provided. **Only the first two answers that you give will be marked** and you will get nothing for a third answer, even if it is correct (this will remain the case even if the first two happen to be incorrect and the last one correct). As a result, it is essential to write down the answers you are most confident of first, up to the number required.

- Some investigations are normally done together and would count as one answer, for instance urea and electrolytes or iron and total iron binding capacity, etc. Others, while commonly done together in a particular disorder (e.g. an electro-cardiogram and echocardiogram, or pulmonary function tests and arterial blood gas tensions), would count as two separate investigations.

7. Understand and answer the question as asked on the paper

- Mistakes can be made, and valuable marks lost, in the paper by reading the question quickly and not being careful to answer what is actually asked.

- Before answering each question, carefully read what answer is required. Have you understood the question? Make sure that you have.

- When asked *"What investigation would you do?"*, having selected your investigations, read the question again very carefully and make sure that you are not repeating any of the investigations that have been given in the question unless it is clinically warranted (e.g. in a patient with a suspected insulinoma, a repeat blood sugar level after fasting would be appropriate even if one normal blood sugar concentration has been given).

8. No negative marking

- Unlike the MCQ paper, wrong answers are not given negative marks. This means that you should attempt **every question**. You therefore need to develop a strategy for making an educated guess.

- If you are not sure of the answer, you can probably widen your chances by being a little less precise. For instance, describing a histological specimen as a *"non-caseating granuloma"* will score more marks than *"granuloma"*, whereas *"caseating granuloma"* will score none. In this situation, if you are not sure which is correct you may get something for *"granuloma"*, but nothing if you are precise and wrong. This is a risky strategy and you should usually try to come to as accurate an answer as you can.

- Towards the end of the written exam you should **go through it again, looking for gaps** where you have not yet written an answer. Even if you consider that the only answer you can think of is extremely unlikely, you must "have a go" and fill the gaps with possibilities. You could be lucky and gain an extra mark or two, and you will certainly not be penalised in any way – no matter how ridiculous your answer may actually be.

Common Questions

Certain topics lend themselves very well to these types of questions. This means that **certain questions come up time and time again**. You should try to spot such areas and commit them to memory, so that they can be easily and reliably reproduced on the day of the exam. Membership books are a useful source for these.

The following is a list of such important areas. You may be able to add to it.

- Tuberculosis and tuberculin testing.
- Acquired immune deficiency syndrome.
- Systemic lupus erythematosus.
- Salmonella.
- Brucellosis.
- Sarcoidosis.
- Hodgkin's disease.
- Fibrosing alveolitis.
- Renal tubular acidosis.
- Porphyrias.
- Malaria and tropical medicine.
- Glucose-6-phosphate dehydrogenase deficiency.
- Sickle cell disease.
- Thalassaemia.

- Cushing's syndrome.

- Lung cancer.

- Bronchopulmonary aspergillosis.

Summary

This is not an easy exam and, if the answers seem obvious, you may have missed the point. Equally you can go to the other extreme and think that every question is a "trick" and miss the obvious or be too clever in your answers. The examiners are attempting to determine your level of knowledge and your ability to process information in a way that is appropriate to the **normal** practice of medicine. The best approach, therefore, is to try to forget that it is an exam and imagine that you are being given this information in an everyday clinical situation. All the information that you are given in the question is important. However, as in routine clinical practice, one item, out of many, may be the key that unlocks the diagnosis, and many others, seemingly relevant, may be "red herrings".

Finally, it is important that you do not get flustered when things do not appear to be going well in the exam room. It is easy, while struggling with a difficult question, to look up and see everyone else apparently busy writing and to assume that you are the only person who is finding it difficult. Provided that you have done your revision adequately, it is likely that if you are finding it difficult so are most of the others in the room. Do not be deceived by their apparent calm; they are probably thinking exactly the same about you. Do not give up or leave the exam part way through. You can still pass even if you do less well on one part of the paper.

Remember that the principles applicable in one section of the written exam may be equally relevant in another; for instance, pictorial and laboratory data may be presented in the clinical cases as well as in the pictorial material and data interpretation sections, respectively. The comments made in each of the following chapters are therefore equally applicable to the others.

Key points

- Time awareness is essential.
- A calm approach is needed.
- Use broad and divergent thinking.
- Take note of the marking system.
- Understand and answer the question as asked.
- Note the number of points requested.
- Think yourself into the clinical situation.
- No negative marking (answer **all** the questions).
- Be **precise** in your answers.
- Practise with lots of case histories, data interpretation and photographic materials.

References

[1] D. J. Weatherall, J. G. G. Leddington and D. A. Warrell, *The Oxford Textbook of Medicine*, 3rd edn, Oxford University Press, Oxford, 1996.
[2] J. Macleod, C. Edwards and I. Bouchier (Ed.), *Davidson's Principles and Practice of Medicine*, 17th edn, Churchill Livingstone, London, 1995.
[3] P. Kumar and M. Clark, *Clinical Medicine*, 3rd edn, Bailliere Tindall, London, 1994.
[4] R. L. Souhami and J. Moxham, *Textbook of Medicine*, Churchill Livingstone, London, 1994.
[5] D. Rubenstein and D. Wayne, *Lecture notes on Clinical Medicine*, Blackwell, Oxford, 1994.
[6] S. R. Meadows and R. W. Smithells, *Lecture notes on Paediatrics*, 6th edn, Blackwell Science, London, 1993.
[7] A. D. Milner and D. Hull, *Hospital Paediatrics*, 2nd edn, Churchill Livingstone, London, 1992.
[8] Medicine International (published yearly). The Medicine Group (UK) Ltd. 62 Stert Street, Abingdon, Oxon OX14 3UQ.
[9] Past Papers are available from the Royal Colleges of Physicians, see Chapter 1.

Chapter 5

Case histories

Introduction

In this part of the exam, which lasts for 55 minutes, you will be presented with four or five case histories and the results of selected investigations. In some cases these will be described, for instance chest X-ray "normal", or you may be given a photograph of a physical sign or investigation. You will then be asked a series of questions.

The principles for effective answering of this part of the exam are similar to those outlined in **Chapter 4**. These will not be repeated fully here, and you must read this chapter in conjunction with the previous one.

The Case History

- Although you may not be asked for the diagnosis, answering questions is much easier if you have correctly understood the problem. Your first aim, therefore, should be to draw up a **list of possible diagnoses** and to rank them according to likelihood based on symptoms, signs and investigations.

- Read the complete question very carefully and **highlight** everything that you think may be important. **Can you see the wood for the trees?**

- Remember that some items of information will hold the key to the diagnosis and others will be "red herrings" (e.g. Cypriot child whose grandmother has tuberculosis and who keeps a parrot raises the possibility of thalassaemia, tuberculosis and psittacosis).

- Even if you think that you have the answer, **still draw up a wide differential diagnosis**. You may find that the results of the investigations you are given make your initial diagnosis unlikely. It is crucial in this situation that you do not press on regardless, but **stop and reconsider**. A classic example is a child who presents with abdominal pain and chickenpox. It is important to consider pneumonia and pancreatitis, but do not forget common causes of abdominal pain in children such as constipation, appendicitis, etc.

- Do not discount a diagnosis or investigation because it seems too simple.

- When going through the investigations you may feel frustrated that you have not been given some information that would normally be available to you and might be very helpful. For instance, you may not be given the result of urea and electrolyte estimations or the full blood count. Unfortunately, there is nothing you can do about this and you must **work with the information that you have been given**.

- Some of the investigation results will exclude, or make very unlikely, diagnoses you have raised as part of your differential diagnosis, and these can then be eliminated. It may also be that the investigations prompt a diagnosis you had not previously considered. You should go through the history again to see whether this fits in with the information you have been given. At this stage it is worth **rewriting** your list of possible diagnoses in order of likelihood.

Answering the Question

You should now turn to the questions. You will be asked to provide one answer or alternatively several answers to a series of related questions. It is very important that you **read these questions carefully and answer them precisely**. You will get no marks for writing the diagnosis, even if it is correct, if you are being asked for the treatment that should be given.

You may be asked to provide:

- A single diagnosis.

- A list of likely diagnoses.

- A further investigation or series of investigations.

- Treatment options.

- An explanation of a symptom or sign.

- An explanation of an abnormal investigation result.

When answering the questions, be as **precise** as possible. For instance, in a patient with a history and cereberospinal fluid findings suggestive of bacterial meningitis you would get more marks for this answer than simply saying "*meningitis*", although this is correct.

If asked for a single investigation, even if you would like to do a battery of tests, you must give only one suggestion. The single investigation that you choose from all those possible will be determined by the information you have been given. This should be the one most likely to yield a **definitive** diagnosis. Sometimes there may be several equally correct answers in which case choose the most relevant initial test.

Example

In a patient with a history and investigations suggestive of renal failure, there are a range of investigations that you could perform.

An estimation of creatinine clearance would be reasonable in all such patients, but is unlikely to score many, if any, marks. If you thought the history was leading you towards a diagnosis of retroperitoneal fibrosis, then computed tomography would be the most appropriate single investigation. If you were suspicious of some form of glomerulonephritis, a renal biopsy would be more appropriate, etc.

If you are not certain, it is best to make a list of all the possible investigations that you could perform and then **rank them** according to which will give you the information most likely to enable you to make a definitive diagnosis.

If you cannot make a definitive diagnosis (and sometimes you will not be able to), then suggest the investigation that you would next do if confronted with this problem in clinical practice. Simple investigations such as *"urea and electrolytes"* may be the correct answer.

If the questions or the results of the investigations do not tally with your diagnosis, do not try to make it all fit your prejudices, but rather reconsider.

Try the following "grey case" using some of the techniques suggested in this chapter.

A Worked Example

A 46-year-old man complained of mild breathlessness on exertion. Three years previously, at a routine assessment performed because of his work in a steel foundry, he was noted to have abnormal spirometry findings and a chest radiograph revealed small-volume lungs. He underwent a drill biopsy of the lung, but this did not yield a suitable specimen for diagnostic purposes. He had four-pillow orthopnoea and found it difficult getting out of his car, but complained of no other symptoms. His father had died at the age of 45 years from a myocardial infarction and a cousin had been confined to a wheelchair since her late thirties. He had smoked 30 cigarettes a day since the age of 17. His hobbies included angling and keeping racing pigeons.

On examination there was no clubbing, chest expansion was reduced and an occasional basal crackle was audible on auscultation. His pulse was 80 beats per minute, the jugular venous pressure (JVP) was not raised and there were no added cardiac sounds or murmurs. He was clearly distressed by breathlessness on lying flat.

Routine haematology and biochemistry were normal. His chest radiograph showed small-volume lungs and the lung fields were generally plethoric. Lung function test results were as follows:

FEV_1	30% predicted
FVC	34% predicted
FEV_1/FVC	91%
Total lung capacity	40% predicted
Residual volume	60% predicted
Transfer factor	62% predicted
Transfer coefficient	110% predicted

1. What is the most likely diagnosis?
2. Suggest two further investigations.

Think about your answers and write them down before reading the worked answer shown.

A possible approach to this question

Go through the question highlighting **anything** that might be relevant.

*A 46-year-old man complained of **mild breathlessness on exertion**. Three years previously, at a routine assessment performed because of his work in a **steel foundry**, he was noted to have **abnormal spirometry** findings and a chest radiograph revealed **small-volume lungs**. He underwent a **drill biopsy** of the lung, but this did not yield a suitable specimen for diagnostic purposes. He had four-pillow **orthopnoea** and found it **difficult getting out of his car**, but complained of no other symptoms. His father had died at the age of 45 years from **myocardial infarction** and a cousin had been **confined to a wheelchair** since her late thirties. He had **smoked** 30 cigarettes a day since the age of 17. His hobbies included angling and keeping **racing pigeons**.*

*On examination there was **no clubbing**, chest expansion was **reduced** and an **occasional basal crackle** was audible on auscultation. His pulse was 80 beats per minute, the **JVP was not raised** and there were **no added cardiac sounds or murmurs**. He was clearly distressed by **breathlessness on lying flat**.*

*Routine haematology and biochemistry were normal. His chest radiograph showed **small-volume lungs** and the lung fields were generally **plethoric**. Lung function test results were as follows:*

FEV$_1$	*30% predicted*
FVC	*34% predicted*
FEV$_1$/FVC	*91%*
Total lung capacity	*40% predicted*
Residual volume	*60% predicted*
Transfer factor	*62% predicted*
Transfer coefficient	*110% predicted*

1. What is the most likely diagnosis?
2. Suggest two further investigations.

From the outset it is clear that the **cardiopulmonary system** is the **focus** of this case. There is a lot of possibly relevant information that throws up a wide differential diagnosis:

(a) The patient worked in a steel foundry – ?some form of occupational lung disease.
(b) He was a heavy smoker – ?obstructive airways disease.
(c) He kept racing pigeons – ?extrinsic allergic alveolitis.
(d) His father died at a young age from a myocardial infarction – could his breathlessness be cardiac in origin?
(e) We are not told why he found it difficult getting out of a car, but it is an unusual symptom to volunteer and **may** be a major clue to the diagnosis – could he have pulmonary fibrosis in association with rheumatoid arthritis?

Let us now consider further each of these:

- Smoking-related obstructive airway disease can be eliminated immediately: the chest radiograph showed small-volume lungs and this is confirmed by the lung function test results, which show a restrictive pattern.

- We are told that he has mild breathlessness on exertion and marked orthopnoea and that he was very uncomfortable lying flat during the examination. This is very suggestive of a **cardiac problem**. However, apart from the family history, which is a rather weak pointer, there is nothing else to suggest cardiac disease. The examination did not reveal any cardiac abnormality. Although we are not told about the heart size on the chest radiograph, there is really nothing to suggest a cardiac problem. Therefore, although we cannot totally exclude this possibility, it seems unlikely at this stage.

- **Could he have pulmonary fibrosis?** He certainly has a number of reasons for having it – his

occupation, his hobbies and the possible rheumatological link – or it could be "cryptogenic".
Someone previously thought he had pulomonary
fibrosis, because they performed a drill biopsy; this
diagnosis would fit with his small-volume lungs
and restrictive lung function test results. **Is there
anything that helps to eliminate any of the
possibilities**? Patients with cryptogenic fibrosing
alveolitis (CFA) are often clubbed and so this is
perhaps less likely, although not impossible.
Secondly, patients with rheumatoid arthritis who
develop pulmonary fibrosis usually have severe
disease and it would not be unreasonable to
expect to be told that he had evidence of arthritis;
the evidence that he does have joint disease is
very circumstantial, namely difficulty getting out of
a car.

So, at this stage, we think that he does not have
smoking-related obstructive airway disease, that
cardiac disease is very unlikely, and that some
form of fibrosis is the most likely, with extrinsic
allergic alveolitis or fibrosis as a consequence of
his work in the steel foundry being the front
runners.

- **Now go back through the history again**. Is there
  anything here that makes pulmonary fibrosis
  unlikely; the answer is "yes". Patients with
  pulmonary fibrosis do not usually complain of
  such marked orthopnoea and, indeed, some are
  more comfortable lying flat. The **mild** breathlessness on exertion and the **marked** increase in
  breathlessness when supine is striking. In addition
  we are told that there is only a very occasional
  crackle. What about the lung function tests? They
  do show a restrictive picture but there are two
  further abnormalities which are surprising in

someone with small lungs due to pulmonary fibrosis. Firstly, the transfer coefficient is **raised**, whereas you would expect it to be reduced and, secondly (this is more subtle and you would not be expected to know this), the residual volume has not fallen by as much as the total lung capacity. **This combination of symptoms and physiology makes any form of pulmonary fibrosis very unlikely**. Unfortunately we are now in the position of having eliminated **all** our possible differentials!

- **Return to the history**. Is there anything else there that we have not yet considered? Why were we told that a **cousin** was confined to a wheelchair? It is unusual to give this in the history unless it is significant. Why might a relative be confined to a wheelchair? The likely possibilities include a joint or neuromuscular problem. We already feel that a joint problem is unlikely but a subtle inherited myopathy could explain his difficulty in getting out of a car. At this point we suddenly remember that we have read somewhere that respiratory muscle weakness can cause orthopnoea and be associated with small-volume lungs. If you are a little more knowledgeable, you will know that it is one of the causes of a **raised** transfer coefficient.

The diagnosis therefore is of respiratory muscle weakness; two further tests would include any of:

- Mouth pressures.
- Electromyography.
- Muscle biopsy.
- Estimation of creatinine phosphokinase level.

The key is to **keep thinking** when your original diagnosis seems unlikely and not to suppress uncomfortable facts which make your answer wrong.

Key points

- Read the questions carefully and answer the question you have been asked.

- Read all the information you are given carefully. One seemingly minor fact may be the key.

- Be as precise and concise as you can.

- Watch out for "red herrings".

- Answer all the questions.

Chapter 6

Data interpretation

Introduction

In this section of the MRCP Part II you will be asked to answer ten questions. The principles for effective answering of this part of the exam are similar to those outlined in **Chapter 4**. These will not be repeated fully here, and you must read this chapter in conjunction with this previous chapter.

Typical Questions

A brief history is usually given followed by some data. These may be:

- Biochemical.
- Haematological.
- Electrocardiographic.
- A dynamic endocrine test.
- Cardiac catheter data.
- Pulmonary function tests.
- Arterial blood gases.
- Viral titres.
- Genetic pedigrees.

Specific Paediatrics topics include:

- Audiograms and tympanograms.
- Electroencephalograms.
- Developmental assessments.
- Picture of chromosomes.

You may be asked to:

- Give a diagnosis.
- Suggest further investigations or treatment.
- Explain symptoms or physical signs that you have been given in the history.

You will be expected to know **normal ranges** for common investigations, but not for less common tests or those in which different normal ranges are in common use (e.g. alkaline phosphatase).

Techniques

- Consider carefully all the information that you have been given and the questions that you have been asked to answer in order to help you respond appropriately.

- Apply common sense and basic principles. You may be able to work it out.

- If you think that you have the correct diagnosis, but cannot think of the required number of further investigations, think again. It is possible that you are on the wrong track.

If you are struggling to provide an answer, the following approach may be helpful:

1. Consider all the **possible diagnoses** that are suggested by the history and physical findings and see whether any of them can be made to tie in with the investigation results.

2. Think of all the **possible conditions** in which you might expect to request the investigations, the results of which you have been given, and see whether this sheds any light on the history given.

3. Consider the possibility of **another event** occurring on the background of **pre-existing disease**, which would explain some unexpected laboratory data (e.g. acute gastrointestinal haemorrhage in a patient with polycythaemia).

- Create your own personalised lists of causes for abnormal investigation results and then see whether you can eliminate some of the diagnostic possibilities. This is illustrated by the case below.

Example

You are presented with some data regarding abnormal calcium levels.

You may be able to work out the answer by considering in turn all the possible abnormalities of calcium homoeostasis that you know. You will be able to eliminate some of these immediately, but others will require more careful thought. This may include:

Common causes:

- Primary hyperparathyroidism.
- Neoplasia.
- Vitamin D toxicity.
- Thiazide diuretics.
- Artefactual (high protein, tourniquet specimen).

Infrequent causes:

- Immobilisation.
- Paget's disease.
- Tertiary hyperparathyroidism.
- Sarcoidosis.
- Hyperthyroidism.

Rare causes:

- Milk alkali syndrome.
- Vitamin A toxicity.
- Addisonian crisis.
- Aluminium toxicity.
- Benign familial hypercalcaemia.

Worked example

The following cardiac catheter data were obtained from an 18-year-old female:

RA	63%	8 mm Hg
RV	63%	100/5
PA	63%	20/5
LA	98%	—
LV	85%	—
Aorta	85%	—

Question: Name three abnormalities.

Try to answer this yourself first. Then turn over the page to see one possible approach which was used by two doctors who had not looked at these sorts of data for several years.

- You do not need to know the normal ranges for saturation or pressure to answer this question, so don't panic if the values seem unfamiliar.

- Start with what you know. Blood is normally deoxygenated in the right side of the heart and oxygenated in the left. The most striking thing, therefore, is the striking drop in saturation that occurs between the left atrium and left ventricle. This must be due to mixing of saturated and desaturated blood. The only explanation for this is a ventriculoseptal defect with a right to left shunt.

- Right to left shunting occurs when the pressure is higher on the right side than the left side of the heart. You have not been given the left-sided pressures, but this is irrelevant.

- A raised pressure on the right side of the heart can be due to an outflow obstruction anywhere from below the pulmonary valve to the left side of the heart.

- Now examine the pressures you have been given. There is a clear step down from the right ventricle to the pulmonary artery. This must be due to an obstruction at or below the pulmonary valve.

- **Using this approach, the answer is pulmonary stenosis with a ventricular septal defect and a right to left shunt.**

An alternative approach is to list every possible anatomical abnormality that might explain abnormal saturation and pressure data. For example, an atrioseptal defect is unlikely because the saturations are appropriate. Eisenmenger's syndrome is unlikely because the pulmonary artery pressures are normal, etc.

Key points

- Time awareness is essential.

- A calm approach is needed.

- Use broad and divergent thinking.

- Take note of the marking system.

- Understand and answer the question as asked.

- Note the number of points requested.

- No negative marking (answer **all** the questions).

- **Practise** lots of data interpretation.

Chapter 7

Photographic material

Introduction

The format of the exam has changed in recent years. You are now provided with printed photographs rather than slides. This allows you to deal quickly with the cases you recognise and leaves more time for the more difficult photographs.

You will be presented with 20 pictures or pairs of pictures. These may include the following:

- Radiographs, radioisotope scans, echocardiograms, magnetic resonance images, computerised tomograms.

- Patients with abnormal physical signs.

- Macroscopic pathology specimens.

- Histological specimens.

- Blood films and bone marrows.

- Retinal photographs.

- Urine samples, for instance showing colour change after a particular test.
- Abnormalities visible to the naked eye in blood samples, e.g. lipaemia.

You may be asked:

- For a diagnosis.

- To provide an explanation of the apparent abnormality.

- To describe associated symptoms or signs.

- To provide a differential diagnosis for the abnormality you can see.

- To suggest further tests or treatment.

For some of the pictures the answer will be obvious immediately, but in others you will have little or no idea of the correct answer. Some of the possibilities that could explain, for instance, an abnormal radiological appearance may not fit with information you have been given in the history. This is similar to clinical practice in which abnormalities in an investigation can be explained by a wide variety of different causes, but the correct answer is indicated by the history.

Example

You are shown a chest radiograph of pulmonary fibrosis.

There is a very wide possible differential diagnosis. However, many of the causes can be eliminated by the occupational, drug or other history. Therefore, if you are asked to provide a possible explanation for the abnormality, this is exactly what you should do, giving the commonest causes first. If the question indicates that you should interpret the investigation in the light of the information given, you will get **no marks** for giving other unrelated possible explanations, **even if they are a correct explanation** of the radiological abnormality. In other words, **read the question carefully**. If in doubt try to tie all your answers in to the others.

Techniques

1. **You may be able to see an abnormality, but not know what it is.**

- Do not give up – lateral thinking is required.

- Read the question again carefully; **are there any hints in the question?**

- Sometimes you may be able to **work out what the picture shows from the information given without even having to look at it**. Think of all the conditions you know which may be associated with abnormalities similar to those that you have been shown. This may jog your memory.

- Remember that it may be something that you have never seen, but have heard described. **Go with your hunches**; if you think *"so that's what it looks like"*, you are probably right.

2. **You may not be able to see an abnormality at all.**

- It is possible that you are being shown something that is normal or a variant of normal. This is certainly possible with radiographs, but is unlikely if you are shown a picture of a patient. See Normals in Ryder *et al.*[1] for useful examples.

- Beware of problems **not associated with an obvious prime pathology**, e.g. always look specifically for gas under the diaphragm, fractures, transposed or reversed radiographs.

- It is worth thinking out before the exam **what you will do** if presented with a picture, of for instance a face or hands, in which you can see no abnormality. Consider all the **subtle abnormalities** that might be seen in pictures of the face or hands respectively, and see whether anything similar is apparent. **Read the background information again: there may be a clue**. For example, if you are given a picture of a blood film and you cannot see any abnormality, the information that the patient had returned from holiday with a fever would prompt you to have a very careful look for malarial parasites, etc.

3. **You may not even know what the picture is of.**

- This is most likely with macroscopic pathology specimens, histology and some radiology.

- The history may help you, but if not, **draw up a shortlist of possible organs** and then list diagnoses for each of these and see whether this brings inspiration.

Example (Figure 1)

It is clear that the child in Fig. 7.1 does not look normal. You may recognise the features as being typical of Down's syndrome. If not, do not make a wild guess. Be less specific: the child is likely to have a chromosomal disorder and the answer may earn you some marks, whereas a specific guess, such as Pierre Robin syndrome, which is wrong would get you none.

Example (Figure 2)

This woman has Raynaud's phenomenon. What is the radiological abnormality? If you cannot see an abnormality

- **Do not panic**.
- Consider what you think the **likely** diagnosis to be from the history and what abnormalities would be expected in the radiology or pathology of that condition.
- Look again at the picture (Fig. 7.2) and see whether you can find any of these abnormalities.

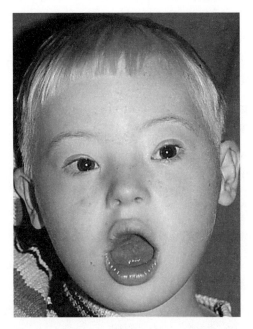

Fig. 7.1 Down's syndrome

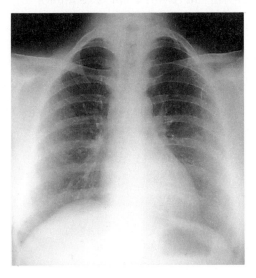

Fig 7.2 A chest radiograph with no apparent abnormality

- **Be systematic**. You know how to read a chest radiograph in a systematic way. Force yourself to do it.

- In particular, examine the apices, behind the heart, the bony thorax, and structures outside the chest.

- Using this approach you are unlikely to miss less obvious abnormalities.

- You will see the abnormality only if you specifically look for it. There is a very small left sided cervical rib.

Key points

- There is no substitute for a broad-based knowledge and understanding.

- Develop the skill of weighing the significance of different "right" answers.

- Practise with lots of photographic materials so that you are familiar with what is required.

- Consider **all** the information you have been given.

- Read the question very carefully.

- Answer as precisely and concisely as you can.

- If you do not know the answer, make a reasoned guess.

Reference

[1] R. E. J. Ryder, M. A. Mir and E. A. Freeman, *An Aid to the MRCP Short Cases*. Blackwell Scientific Publications, Oxford, 1996.

Part III

The clinical exams

Chapter 8

After the written exam

Introduction

Many people sit the MRCP exams, yet less than half the candidates pass each time. To pass the exam as a whole, you **must** be successful in the clinical exam and cannot fail any section outright. Do not wait for the results of the written exam before turning your attention to preparing for the clinical exam. After sitting the written exam it can certainly help to have the weekend off studying to recharge your batteries. After this, you must then get back to the work of passing the clinical exams.

There are generally about 6–8 weeks between the two exams. Thorough preparation for the clinical exam is essential but often neglected. You would not dream of sitting your driving test by reading the highway code and not practising your driving for the driving test. The clinical exam is totally different from the written one and requires you to have an excellent factual knowledge which you must be able to apply clinically. Spend the next 6–8 weeks learning how to present your answers effectively.

How to Prepare

- Regular practice at answering questions will significantly improve your ability to structure and present answers.

- It is very difficult to prepare adequately for the clinical exam completely by yourself. Consider working with a **group** of candidates who are applying for the same exam. Organise teaching opportunities for the entire group. Studying as part of a group allows mutual motivation and also enables you to compare your level of knowledge with that of others.

- The more clinical teaching the better. Take every opportunity to practise presenting and answering questions.

Revision strategy for the clinical

Use your job to help you revise. Treat every patient that you see in Casualty and Outpatients as a potential Long Case. Try not to read the general practitioner's referral letter first, but approach the case afresh. For example, if asked to see someone with chest pain, assess the patient first before looking at the electrocardiogram. Similarly, if asked to see someone with pneumonia, examine the patient before looking at the chest radiograph. Always take a good social history and think through how your patient's illness will affect them.

How can you stand out as being someone who should pass?

The general principles of doing well in the clinical exams are to organise your knowledge, making sure that what you say is:

- Clear.

- Relevant.

- Interesting.

Remember that the purpose of the exam is to identify a safe, competent and professional registrar. It is more important to have a solid grasp of the basic principles of treatment than the fine detail. Previous candidates will claim that they failed for all sorts of trivial reasons. One candidate claimed she failed because she did not know which component of house-dust mite faeces was responsible for exacerbating asthma. Rumours like this are frequent and may be spread by previous unsuccessful candidates. Do not allow them to reduce your confidence or commitment to pass.

Remember

- You have done this all before.
- Clear communicators consistently do well in the clinical.
- **You are presenting yourself** not merely the case.
- You are also being asked to demonstrate your skills as a clinician.

Structure of the Clinical Exam

There are three parts to the clinical exams:

- The Long Case.
- The Short Cases.
- The Viva/oral.

At the start of the exam you will be given three personalised examination sheets. You must submit these in turn during each part of the exam to the examiners. For each section of the exam there will be two examiners, making six in all. The examiners will alternate between asking questions and marking your answers.

- **The Long Case** examination involves a period of 1 hour with the patient followed by an interview lasting 20 minutes with two examiners. They will ask questions relating to the diagnosis, history, examination, possible investigations, planned management and prognosis. Usually only one examiner will ask the questions. Both examiners will mark independently and then agree on a final mark. They may take you back to the patient and ask you to demonstrate a clinical sign you have described.

- **The Short Cases** last 30 minutes, and a variable number of cases will be seen. There is no fixed number of cases that you must complete in order to pass. People have passed (and failed) with as few as three cases, or as many as ten or more. The examiners have 15 minutes each to ask questions. Each marks independently and then agree on a final joint mark.

- **The Viva** lasts 20 minutes, with two further examiners. In most centres all three sections of the exam will follow one after another. In hospitals near to the Royal Colleges (Glasgow, Edinburgh and London), the Viva may be held in the College itself.

Coming to the Exam

Think

- What will I wear?

- What impression do I want to give? (clothes, haircut, etc.)

- What will I do over the lunchtime break? (Do not smell of alcohol, smoke, garlic or curry!)

How can I arrive on time?

It is surprising how often this causes problems. Expect the unexpected (traffic jams, rail strikes, losing your car keys, etc.). **If you are late for any part of the exam it will leave you feeling tense, pressured and unlikely to perform well**. It can destroy months of hard work, and mean that you will have to repeat all your revision once again. Definitely consider staying overnight in a **nice** hotel (not noisy). It is worth the money. Some hotels offer reduced rates for MRCP candidates; others may offer corporate rates for your hospital Trust. A long drive with an early start can seem too far on the actual day and will leave you feeling stressed. You will probably not have slept well and being "on-site" can make a big difference.

The following three chapters go through each aspect of the clinical exams. Do not try to learn the suggestions off by heart. Instead, you will find the chapters of most help if you integrate those areas you find most helpful into your current approach. **Never change your style of presenting on the day**. You must seek to adopt an approach to the exams which is well learned and practised. Adapt the techniques for yourself, and seek honest (and constructive) feedback from others.

Key points

- The clinical is in three parts: Long Case, Short Cases and the Viva.

- You will be examined by three pairs of examiners.

- You are presenting yourself, not just the case.

- Look smart and professional.

- Arrive early. Consider staying in a quiet hotel close to the exam venue.

- Do not try radically to change your presentation techniques on the day.

Chapter 9

The Long Case

Preparing for the Long Case

The **long case is the part of the exam nearest to clinical practice** as a hospital physician. The best environment to learn this is therefore a busy general medical job and the relevant specialties in order that you become familiar with established practice. No amount of book reading will make up for a deficit in clinical awareness and the skills gained in the day-to-day practice of medicine. During your senior house officer years, you should learn from your seniors and take the opportunity to discuss the **reasoning behind the investigation and management of the patients under your care** (this includes radiologists and other specialists). Merely carrying out a list of duties each day will be both unrewarding and uneducational. Each new patient can potentially be tackled with the same enthusiasm as the exam Long Case and you should make it the norm to **commit yourself to a differential diagnosis, investigation plan and management strategy**. Only by doing this **regularly** will you improve your examination performance and, more importantly, your clinical practice. The Long Case aims to test your abilities as an effective and competent clinician. The examiners' key question is "**Would I be happy with you as my registrar**". You need to convey an impression of reliability and safety. In the same way that in a driving test you need to make the instructor feel safe while you drive, in these exams you need to show the examiners that you are a safe, sensible and competent

---

clinician who could be trusted to look after their patients. You must therefore communicate in your presentation that you are:

- Safe.

- Sensible.

- Competent.

- Professional.

In each section of the Part II exam the examiners mark your answers **separately**, and then compare their independent marks in order to decide on a **final agreed joint mark** which is submitted to the College.

To prepare

- Practise presenting cases.

- Seek out opportunities to present cases at staff rounds, etc.; these will give you practice at answering unexpected questions under pressure.

- Seek supervised training in presentation skills. **Watch yourself presenting on video**. This is the most effective way of changing. It has the added advantage that the actual exam will be no more stressful than this.

Mock Long Case Exams

In addition to learning through your general clinical work, you should also seek specific experience in all parts of the exam. The Short Cases are usually thought of in this teaching frame, but practice with the Long Case is equally important.

Ask your seniors, and your consultants especially, if you can present Long Cases to them on a more formal basis. Most of them will oblige if asked at the correct moment.

If there are any Part II clinical examiners at your hospital, try to arrange a mock clinical with them. Be willing to accept their feedback and suggestions to change. Ultimately, however, you are seeking to develop a clinical interview and presentation style with which **you** are happy.

It is best to gain experience in being examined by a range of different people who have different personal styles of examining. Do not omit practice with examiners who are regarded as "hard". This can be an invaluable experience, although it is probably best to avoid having such a mock examiner for your last practice before the exams - this could have an unhelpful impact on morale.

In all mock exams, try to seek **specific and constructive feedback**. A feedback sheet such as the assessment sheet shown below can help form the basis for this. Do not accept all feedback at face value: are the comments accurate, helpful and balanced? If not, seek a further opinion.

It can be quite difficult to make yourself practise in this way. Some find that presenting to a group of other colleagues who are also sitting the exam can be helpful. You will gain from seeing how others present their cases, and they will also learn from you.

Try presenting the cases to each other using the formal approach of presenting to two "examiners" as in the exam. Try to present a patient who is under the care of a colleague, to someone not directly involved with the case. This prevents them asking you unfairly about information that they know from outside the examination setting.

Ask friends working in other hospitals to show you their interesting or challenging cases. In your own hospital, you may realise that this is the patient with the enlarged spleen that your colleagues were talking about over lunch!

If you work in a very specialised area, you must make sure that you obtain experience with a wide range of general cases. The reverse is also true. It can be helpful to see patients who are being cared for by specialist teams. Obtain varied experience and clinical training in the jobs you choose.

Mock clinical exam assessment sheet

Examiner: **Candidate:**

Initial case presentation:
The ability to pick out the salient features of the case and present these clearly and coherently is stressed. The organisation of information is particularly important. The assessment of relevant physical factors should be recognised in the mark.

Professionalism:
Politeness and professional attitude. The ability to cover the appropriate clinical areas quickly, clearly and efficiently.

Discussion of the differential diagnosis, aetiology, management and prognosis of the case:
Paying regard to social and psychological factors as well as purely physical approaches.

Overall mark:
A general discussion with the candidate would probably be the most help rather than an overall statement of Pass or Fail.

Comments:
Helpful ways to improve presentation and organisation of material.

(Please photocopy and use if you wish.)

Mock Clinical Exams

Make sure that you do mock clinical exams in each of the main areas of clinical practice. The following disorders are common in practice, and hence are common in exams:

- Cardiac.
- Neurological.

- Respiratory.
- Gastroenterological.
- Haematological.
- Rheumatological
- Renal.

Predicting and Practising Cases

Try to remember that the hospital where you sit the examination will tend to have the same types of patient that you see in your own clinical practice. The hospital has to provide approximately 20–30 patients for the Long Cases and these are therefore likely to include both inpatients and outpatients. Many find it useful either to write down full assessment and management plans of a "typical" case, or to test and be tested by peers who are also taking the exam. However, **do not just regurgitate prepared lists** in the exam – remember that every patient is an individual and each case is different. Do not be put off if your findings do not quite "fit" or are not "typical". Common conditions may have atypical features.

Even mock exams are stressful, but you are far better off learning from your mistakes **before** rather than in the heat of the exam when you have paid your money and made it through the written exam. Knowing you have an effective presentation style can help to lower your anxiety in the exam setting. Try to practise presenting in stressful situations (e.g. in front of others or to the professor). It will make the exam itself seem less stressful.

Write out full assessment and management plans for each of the following: (Be able to present these concisely and efficiently in an informed manner.)

- Heart failure, hypertension, myocardial infarction and ischaemic heart disease.

- Renal failure.

- Asthma.

- Any area that the examining hospital is known to specialise in.

- Know about current controversies (e.g. the use of regular beta-agonists in asthma).

- Familiarise yourself with local accents and dialects, particularly if English is not your first language.

Do not attempt to visit or contact the clinical staff or wards of the hospital at which you will be examined. This can lead to you being disqualified from the exam.

The overriding thing to have in mind is that the patients chosen for the exams will be **appropriate** for the level of exam you are sitting. Sometimes the patient's condition may seem very complex. You can still pass the exam by keeping calm and concentrating on technique.

On the Day

There is a great temptation to carry everything you may ever need into the clinical exam. All this will achieve is a set of heavy pockets and the impression of a clumsy, nervous candidate who will undoubtedly leave something behind during the course of the exam. The job of the Registrar at the examining centre is to remove this burden of responsibility for equipment and **to provide the necessary tools** at the correct time and place. (There have been many candidates turn up with red and white hat pins but no stethoscope.)

Essentials:

- A smart professional appearance.

- A pen that works, plus a spare.

- A highlighter or red pen can be useful.

- Stethoscope.

- Watch with second hand.

- Pen torch.

- Orange sticks (plantar reflexes and pinprick testing when broken).

- Red hat pin for central scotoma and colour vision. (This is not advisable on the Paediatric exam.)

Non-essentials (provided by examination centre):

- Ophthalmoscope.

- Tendon hammer.

- Snellen chart.

- Reading material (visual acuity at bedside).

- Cotton wool (corneal reflexes and light touch).

- Tuning fork.

- Tongue depressor.

- Measuring tape.

- Urine dipsticks.

Winning Over the Patient

- Introduce yourself properly to the patient, and always **address** them formally by their **surname** unless the patient specifies otherwise. (Even so, always by their surname in front of the examiners.)

- The **patients** should **have been instructed to divulge all they know of their condition**, and the more relaxed they are, the better able they will be to help you.

- Explain what you are going to do, and why. Gaining the confidence of the patient is half the battle. They will certainly be aware that the average candidate is nervous and are invariably keen to help you through the exam.

- Explain that you need to take some notes to help you remember.

- **Apologise** in advance for having to interrupt them; say why (it is an exam; time pressures, etc.).

- When you do interrupt, say something like "*I'm sorry to interrupt you again, but I need to ask . . .* "

- Be polite and professional.

- **Don't panic** if it seems to be a very complex case. The examiners know this and will make allowances.

Remain **polite and courteous at all times** but try to be firm in order to **keep to time**.

It is a good idea to spell out your **intended schedule** to the patient from the outset. Tell them that you will initially talk about their illness for approximately 20 minutes and then will move on to the physical examination (further 20 minutes). You will then **recap the main points** with the patient and spend the last 10–15 minutes making some additional notes (differential diagnosis, investigations and management plan). Point out that if there is anything relevant that you may have overlooked they should not hesitate to make you aware of the omission. While making your final notes, the patient is still at hand for those last minute questions.

Remember, even a nervous smile can disarm a tense situation.

Organisation in History Taking

Examiners do not know very much information about the patient you have seen. All they see is a basic written summary from the Senior House Officer or Registrar looking after the patient. What you need to do is **paint a picture** of the patient for them. To present this clearly to the examiners it is vital to **cluster symptoms together logically while taking the history, and therefore while presenting**. This is the key to a good presentation.

- Allow the patient to start to convey the history without initial interruption. You will obviously have to **guide the interview** but it helps to get the patient talking in order to reveal the relevant topic early.

- Make sure you cover all the areas, and impose a clear structure on what you do. Do not allow yourself to be distracted off the task in hand by the patient. You have studied too long and hard to allow this to happen.

- Once the Presenting Complaint is established, it is a good idea to make a note of the possible differ-ential diagnoses, even at this stage. This enables you to **target your interview and seek positive and negative evidence for and against your ultimate diagnosis**.

- The Past Medical History is important not only in

relation to the Presenting Complaint but should also remind you to look for any stigmata of these previous events when examining the patient.

- A thorough Social History is necessary to tailor your management plan, but it is also true that many an examiner will turn to the Social History when the questions dry up, so be prepared. The impact of illness on the patient, their family and work is increasingly important in the MRCP examinations.[1] Make sure you briefly ask about:

1. How their illness is **affecting them** (emotionally).
2. How they are **coping** with their illness.
3. Enquire if they ever feel **worried or depressed** about things.
4. How does their illness **affect their daily life** (e.g. shopping, cooking, getting upstairs).

Techniques Used in the Patient Examination

Nothing creates an impression of disorganisation more than a flurry of paper during the presentation. This can be reduced by a few simple techniques:

- **Extensive note taking is not required** and you should concentrate on the main points.

- **Leave gaps** between each area on your history sheets. You **will** forget questions and this allows you to fit in later questions without creating an unreadable mass of extra notes scribbled in margins.

- You can always **ask the patient** what diagnosis they have been given, and also what treatments or investigations they have had. This can offer very useful clues.

- **Maintain momentum**. You cannot afford to run out of time.

- Aim to finish in 45 minutes. Ask the patient to stay.

- Write on only one side of the paper.

- Number the sheets.

- Organise your information clearly as you take the history.

- Use clear headings (Presenting Complaint, Social History, etc.).

- Consider **writing the headings down** at the start of the exam. This can help you pace your history taking, and also prevents you forgetting to ask about any central and important area.

- Show empathy and concern.

- Show the patient that you are interested in how they are as a person and not just their physical pathology.

Organisation in the Examination

- **Take the patient's blood pressure first**, so that it is not forgotten or missed out as a result of lack of time later.

- Perform a thorough **examination of the primary system related to the presenting complaint**.

- A swift professional **general examination should cover all systems** but look particularly for signs of **complications** of the primary disorder and for **evidence corroborating** your diagnosis.

- If there is **anything obvious** evident (e.g. a leg prosthesis), **make sure you say it**. It is surprisingly common to omit stating the obvious.

- **Remember the urine dipstick**. Do learn how to do this before the day. It may be necessary to read the instructions if you are asked to use a brand with which you are not familiar.

- Internal examinations are not to be performed in the exam.

While taking the history, use a style most examiners will recognise. This is outlined in all basic textbooks of medicine and clinical examination:[2]

- Presenting complaint/history of presenting complaint (PC/HPC).
- Review of systems.
- Past medical history.
- Family history (FH).
- Social history.
- Drugs/allergies.
- Relevant findings from the physical examination.

The Vital Quarter Hour

Taking some time to **collect your thoughts** and yet still have access to the patient is essential. Try to finish your initial history and examination with 15 minutes to go. Don't let the patient leave. Go through your notes again. You will have forgotten to ask about some aspect of the history, or the physical examination, and this is the chance to clarify these.

The good news is that you know in advance what areas the examiners are likely to ask. You will be asked to present your case summary, including the key physical findings, justify your differential diagnosis, and discuss possible investigation and management plans. Think about likely questions from the examiners. Have you sufficient information to answer them?

Read back your case summary to the patient to see whether they agree that this is accurate and summarises the main problems effectively. This can help prevent the embarrassment of the patient changing their story the moment you are examined.

The history may have changed since it was written for the examiners, or the patient may now be partially treated or have relapsed. It is quite reasonable to say this, and this further shows that you are thoughtful and clinically astute. Also, remember the clinical effects of medication on the presentation.

Time at the end of the Long Case allows you to **commit yourself to a differential diagnosis** and to think through your reasons for and against each of the possible diagnoses.

In essence, the Long Case in the **MRCP exam is testing your ability to formulate an investigation and effective management plan** having collected the relevant information from the patient. The last 10–15 minutes with the patient should be used with this aim in mind.

- Read through your notes, and consider using a **red pen** to highlight important areas which you will mention in the presentation. A highlighter pen may also be useful for this purpose.

- Think about writing out your opening sentence. A good start to the presentation can help calm the nerves and offer the right impression.

You have approximately 7–10 minutes to present the whole case. Of this, **it is the opening few minutes that matter the most**. It is during this time that you will present either a favourable or unfavourable impression of yourself. Examiners, being human, tend to label you as clearly passing or failing early in the presentation. In our experience, it is quite difficult to switch between these labels once they are applied; therefore it is vital to have the "right" label attached as soon as possible. How can you make this happen?

Think through your opening few sentences. If the patient has been a difficult or poor historian, say so now and possibly again later, but only once more. Do not overstate this.

- Finally, thank the patient and mention that you may be asked to examine them again in front of the examiners.

Presenting to the Examiners

- Make sure the pages of your history are in the correct order. Fold up your summary and place it in your pocket. Once you have been introduced to the examiners and have sat down, you can safely retrieve it as an aide memoire. **Do not read verbatim from your notes. Instead, try to create your presentation from the key words you have highlighted earlier.**

- Smile. Try to make appropriate eye contact at an early point.

- Be careful to **listen to the question** you have been asked and not to leap into a recital of the full history and examination.

- Although only one examiner will be asking questions at any time, you should answer to both examiners since it is the other examiner who is marking you on that question.

- Be prepared to be interrupted. Examiners are asked

not to let the candidate recite a full history, but instead to pursue problem-orientated questions.

- If asked for a summary, **present the case as though you were the registrar** on the consultant's ward round.

- Can you see the wood for the trees? Present the key findings and salient features of the case.

- Do not be worried if a third examiner is sitting in the background. He or she is a trainee examiner. They will make no contribution at all to your final mark, which is decided by the other two examiners alone.

- Be polite to the examiners, but do not come over as too eager to please. Too much obsequience and the use of "sir" is unwise.

Have ready:

- The relevant positive and negative findings in the history.

- Your differential diagnosis and the reasons for this.

- Your planned investigations.

- Your planned management.

- An estimate of prognosis.

- What you would tell the patient.

- Possible complications of your diagnosis and treatment.

Relevant findings and the differential diagnosis

A pathological classification of disease states provides the structure of our learning at medical school. A diagnostic approach based on symptoms and signs is nearer to working practice. You must first cast your net wide over all possible diagnoses and then progressively eliminate some and confirm others. A number of techniques can be used to help this.

1. The "anatomical sieve"

Is the problem due to a superficial or a deep structure? For example, chest pain may result from a variety of sources:

- Cardiac (ischaemic, pericarditis).
- Pulmonary (embolism, pneumonia).
- Musculoskeletal or connective tissue.
- Oesophageal.
- Tumour.
- Dissecting aortic aneurysm.
- Other.

Another way is to group this into **organ systems** (e.g. renal, pre-renal, post-renal, etc.).

2. The "surgical sieve"

When faced with a lesion, consider its possible aetiology using the following questions. Is it:

- Inherited.
- Congenital.
- Metabolic.
- Infective.

- Inflammatory.
- Vascular.
- Neoplastic.
- Toxin or drug.
- Degenerative.
- Traumatic.
- Nutritional.
- Other.

Overlay the surgical sieve over the anatomical sieve in order to use this approach most effectively.

Try this technique for yourself.

Example

Causes of haematoproteinuria can include:

Spend a few minutes considering this and writing down your answers. A possible answer is provided below.

Possible answer:

Causes of haematoproteinuria include:

Pre-renal:
- Inherited (haemophilia).
- Infective (subacute bacterial endocarditis, etc.).
- Vascular (hypertension, etc.).

Renal:
- Inherited (polycystic kidneys, Alport's syndrome, etc.).
- Congenital (reflux nephropathy, etc.).
- Metabolic (diabetes mellitus, hyperuricaemia, etc.).
- Infective (tuberculosis, urinary tract infection, etc.).

- Inflammatory (systemic lupus erythematosus, polyarteritis nodosa, etc.).

- Vascular (arteriovenous malformation, etc.).

- Neoplastic (renal cell carcinoma, non-metastatic membranous nephropathy, etc.).

- Toxin or drug (non-steroidal anti-inflammatory drugs, penicillamine, etc.).

Post-renal:
- Congenital (spinal bifida with collecting system abnormalities, etc.).

- Metabolic (renal stones, etc.).

- Infective (urinary tract infection, cystitis, pyelonephritis, etc.).

- Inflammatory (retroperitoneal fibrosis, etc.).

- Neoplastic (urothelial tumours or invading tumours, etc.).

- Toxin or drug (cyclophosphamide, etc.).

This illustrates the sort of answer that can be given. It is neither exclusive nor an example of perfection. Ultimately, you must present your own answer in your own words.

Target your presentation specifically to confirm or exclude each of your differential diagnoses by querying the presence or absence of associated symptoms and, later in the examination, the signs. The pain of pericarditis for instance is described as a dull pain with sharp exacerbations associated with lying flat or breathing. It is not related to exertion but the patient may be unable to take a deep breath. It may occur with a fever and recent viral prodrome or post-myocardial infarction. The patient is unlikely to have had it before unless a systemic disorder is the cause (i.e. systemic lupus erythematosus). It can occur in association with pulmonary embolism or pneumonia involving lung parenchyma which abuts on to the pericardium.

You need to communicate to the examiners that you have **considered all relevant diagnostic factors** in your assessment. When you present your findings or diagnosis you should therefore back it up with the reasoning behind your conclusion.

You must not give a category from the surgical sieve if you do not have an example to hand.

When presenting the differential diagnosis, remember that:

- There may be **no single right answer**.

- *"There are a number of possibilities which include . . ."*

- If it is obvious, state what you consider the diagnosis to be.

- Show that you know patients can change, and that your opinions are not fixed but are based on the evidence that you find **now** at interview.

- The examiners' summary of the case includes only **key relevant details**. Do not automatically assume that they have some vital piece of information that you have not discovered. It is important to remember that you will know far more details than the examiners.

If the case is very complicated, don't panic. Instead you can use a phrase such as:

*"This is a very complicated case. After an hour with the patient and without the chance to review the old notes or investigations, I have a **range** of differential diagnoses, but at the present time I would not be able to put them into any definite order. However, my differential diagnosis at present is . . ."*

State the diagnosis you favour at the present time. Using information from the history, make the case **for and against** each of the differential diagnoses in turn.

"Standardised" differential diagnoses

It can be very helpful to have pre-prepared a list of "standardised" differential diagnoses for the common presenting complaints that you come across. These are not lists merely to regurgitate in exams, but instead help you to remember the **range of diagnostic possibilities**. Having these to fall back on can be a great help if anxiety levels are high and you are finding it difficult to think effectively during the exam. Do remember to state these only if you **really are** considering them for this particular case. Create your own "standardised differential diagnoses" for a range of common presentations.

Remember to consider the full range of **physical and psychiatric factors** that may present. For example, conditions such as gastric cancer may obviously present with weight loss, but so too can depression. It can be seen, therefore, that psychiatric diagnoses can present with "physical" complaints, although these are less common in the exam. It is more common in the exam to be asked about ways in which psychological factors affect how the person copes with their illness.

Investigations

Start with **simple tests** first which can be **performed at the bedside** (examination of sputum, peak expiratory flow rate, temperature pulse and respiration chart, etc.). Avoid responding to every question with "*I would take a full history and examination*". This will annoy the examiners. They know you have already seen and assessed the patient.

Think in advance about which other investigations are **appropriate** for each illness. "*These could include . . .*":

- **Laboratory tests** that are likely to be easily available. State **which and why**. Know **what these are done for** and the relevance if they reveal an abnormality (e.g. full blood count to exclude the possibility of anaemia, etc.).

- **Simple radiological tests** (chest X-ray) if appropriate.

- Move on to **confirmatory tests** (full spirometry, bronchoscopy, computerised tomography of the chest, etc.).

- You may be asked early for a specific **definitive test** (e.g. transbronchial lung biopsy for *Pneumocystis carinii*).

Use common sense. Say what you do in **practice**.

Management plans

- Remember what the patient sees as the main problem and ensure that you take account of this.

- If asked what your **immediate management on admission** of a patient would be, start with the steps necessary to ensure the **patient's immediate safety** as if you were the duty resident medical officer (**A**irway, **B**reathing, **C**irculation, if appropriate).

- Say simple things first. For example, you would offer **supportive measures** for a patient with heart failure such as sitting them upright in bed and commencing oxygen therapy.

- Simple measures include **relevant communications to the nursing staff** or other ward professionals to investigate the patient's mobility, observations, fluid intake, diet, etc.

- **Medical intervention with drugs** (i.e. intravenous loop diuretic followed by regular oral diuretics and commencement of medication such as angiotensin converting enzyme inhibitors for heart failure).

- **Non-pharmacological intervention** (i.e. angioplasty or balloon valvotomy).

- **Surgical interventions** (e.g. mitral valve replacement).

- **Rehabilitation** (physical, social, psychological and spiritual, and financial – free prescriptions for diabetics).

- The **specialist opinion** of a doctor in another specialty may be indicated. Requesting an assessment by a physiotherapist or occupational therapist may sometimes also be helpful in the assessment and treatment of the patient.

- **Information giving**. Education, instructions and advice to the patient and their relatives may be important.

- **Timing of discharge** from hospital if an inpatient.

- The illness may not only have biological implications but may result in a change in home, occupation or financial security, for instance.

- A **planned discharge**. Additional **support in the community** may be required. This may include referral for district nurse, hospice, social services, Macmillan nurses, etc.

- Indicate what you might **tell the patient or family** if asked about the possible outcome relating to this illness.

- **Support** for the patient and their family is always important, particularly in chronic or life-threatening presentations.

Prognosis

State your experience, not just papers. Consider:

1. **The classical prognosis of this condition.**
2. **Specific features of this patient that affect the case**.

- Previous history.

- Response to medication.

- Compliance with treatment.

- Social support.

- Characteristics and personality strengths of the patient.

- Try to give the important indicators for a good or bad prognosis in the patient you have seen.

- Emphasise that, because of the prognosis, your treatment is symptomatic, supportive or curative.

Summary

The Long Case needs as much attention as the Short Cases in your preparation. You must develop a technique of interview, examination and presentation which is second nature. You should not change this on the day of the exam. A professional courteous manner is important. Remember you are presenting yourself as well as the case. Be prepared to discuss a summary of your findings with particular reference to relevant positive and negative findings. The diagnosis, differential diagnosis, investigations and management plan will be the subject of the examiners' questions, and the vital quarter hour should be used with this in mind.

Key points

The exam involves:

- Meeting a patient for the first time and winning his/her confidence.

- Obtaining a fully structured and relevant history.

- The physical examination, which concentrates especially on areas that will aid in establishing a diagnosis and confirming or excluding the presence of any complications of the condition.

- Not neglecting the assessment of relevant psychological and social problems.

- Planning your investigations and management according to the differential diagnosis.

- Making sure that you come over as safe, sensible and professional.

- Trying to answer as if this was an everyday clinical situation.

References

[1] Royal Colleges of Physicians and Psychiatrists, *Joint Working Party Report: The Psychological Care of Medical Patients: Recognition of Need and Service Provision*, Royal College of Physicians: London.
[2] J. Munro and C. Edwards (eds) *MacLeod's Clinical Examination*, 8th edn, Churchill Livingstone, London, 1990.

Chapter 10

The Short Cases

Preparing for the Short Cases

For many candidates the Short Cases appear to offer the greatest hurdle to be overcome. Even those with good clinical skills and knowledge may experience difficulty with this part of the exam. Preparation is vital, particularly with practice under examination conditions.

The Short Cases test your breadth of knowledge and your ability to jump from one system to the next as you would have to in casualty, where one moment you may be dealing with acute left ventricular failure and the next with a case of transverse myelitis. They can involve anything from an end-of-the-bed spot diagnosis, to a full neurological examination or assessment of higher intellectual function. All of these are within the capability of most doctors sitting the MRCP examination, but the key is to be able to **perform them whilst under pressure**, in the presence of the examiners, and to look like you have done it a thousand times before. The exam is not the place to do this for the first time. **Your technique must be second nature**. The examination must flow naturally, briskly and be thorough. This leaves your mind clear to concentrate on the findings and differential diagnosis. Being able to think while you work will mean you can look for the confirmatory signs or associated findings that put you one step ahead.

Short Case practice and mock exams

- **Each new patient** you see when working provides **an opportunity to practise**. This will improve your technique and refine your clinical skills. It will only look like second nature when it is second nature.

- Try to identify your clinical and academic **"blindspots"**. Each of us has areas of clinical skills and knowledge that are less strong than other areas. Try to identify these, and work at improving them to at least a reasonable level.

- **Form a peer teaching group** with other colleagues who are also sitting the exam.

- **Arrange a regular session** when you all meet and show each other the exam-oriented cases you have on the wards.

- **Find** as many **"friendly" registrars and senior registrars** as you can and seek regular exam practice. It is best to spread the work out between them. Producing a printed timetable can help this.

- **Limit the number of participants at each teaching session** to avoid an unmanageable and intimidating group.

- The sessions provide an opportunity for fine tuning examination technique, and also short sharp questioning to help you answer whilst under pressure and scrutiny. You need to be able to **substantiate your findings** and differential diagnosis.

- **Consultants are** more difficult to come by, but are **"value for money"** if they can be talked into it. Some of them may even be college examiners, and practice with them is definitely worthwhile. They can offer useful additional comments on the structure and content of your presentations.

Courses

A lot of short cases are outpatients who are brought to the hospital specifically for the examination. If you cannot get to see a wide range of "**classic**" cases in your clinical job, then a clinical course may be helpful. Most hospitals are now running their own courses and many are advertised frequently in the major medical journals.

Techniques

- Go in and act confidently.

- Passing the clinical is a presentation of yourself.

- Do not say your name. Hand over your personalised **examination sheet** when asked.

- Shake the examiners' hands if they initiate this.

- Smile and try to remember the examiners' names. You can then introduce them quickly to the patients.

- Look professional and act competently.

- Be polite but do not come over as too eager to please.

- Make eye contact with both examiners as you start presenting, **and** subsequently.

- Avoid looking at the floor if you don't know something. If the examiners enquire about something that you have forgotten about, say that you would *normally have enquired about this but have forgotten to, and why it would be important* **in this case**.

- Try to appear human by showing (positive) aspects of your personality.

- Be clear and confident.

- **Be interesting**.

- Listen very carefully to the question: do what is asked, and then repeat back to the examiner what has been seen, felt and heard. From these pieces of factual information the candidate needs to suggest a diagnosis.

- You may gain marks by indicating features that are not present and which could have been expected to be present but are absent. For example, *"in the fundus I see retinal haemorrhages, hard and soft exudates, neovascularisation, but no microaneurysms"*. Such a reply indicates to the examiner that the candidate knows the features of diabetic retinopathy, but in addition, knows that not all features need to be present to make the diagnosis.

- It is very rare for the examiners to ask for a spot diagnosis.

Approach to the patient

- **Remain formal and polite**. Always introduce yourself properly to each patient before proceeding. Ask if you may perform the examination asked of you by the examiners.

- Talk to the patient in the way that you normally would. Would you normally address them as "sir" or "madam" six times while examining the cranial nerves? Avoid over-familiarity. Do not use first names – this will annoy some examiners.

- **Show concern for the patient's comfort.**

- **Position the patient** correctly for the particular examination you will carry out (45 degrees for a cardiovascular examination).

- **Enquire whether the patient has any pain before proceeding.** This may target your approach and enables you to be seen to be compassionate in avoiding unnecessary discomfort to the patient.

- **After the examination** of each patient is complete, ensure the patient is again comfortable and **offer to help replace any items of clothing** you may have removed for the examination.

- The key is to be **calm, respectful, considerate and professional.**

It is also important to be adaptable and flexible. Consider carefully any suggestions the examiners make to you about diagnosis, etc. **Do not reject this out of hand**, but show that you can consider the relative evidence for and against a particular diagnostic possibility. If what they say throws you, remember (and tell the examiners) that all you can comment on is the evidence that you found during your examination. **Never** guess – it is better to admit that you cannot hear a diastolic murmur, but to show that you know how to position the patient properly to maximise your chances of hearing it, than just to make a wild guess. **The examiners are not interested in guesses**, even if they happen to be right, but are looking for a professional and competent approach.

Museum cases

The Royal College advises participating hospitals against using so-called classic "museum cases" in the MRCP examination and prefers to use cases that test the candidate's clinical skills rather than their recall for the outstandingly obscure. If you do come across a rarity, then keep calm and work from common sense and first principles. You cannot be expected to have seen everything before but must be able to remain logical. Using effective and well-practised examination techniques can help you come through this safely.

On the Day

All necessary equipment will be provided at the correct time and in the correct place (see the Long Case chapter for what you need on the day).

- Many candidates worry excessively about fundoscopy. A working ophthalmoscope is provided at the examination centre and the relevant Short Cases should be in a darkened room with their pupils dilated by appropriate drops before your arrival.

- It is important that you can use an ophthalmoscope effectively. Make sure you can describe and diagnose the range of intraocular pathology that may present – particularly chronic disorders such as optic atrophy, diabetic and hypertensive retinopathy.

What to do when asked a question

When asked to perform an examination, **listen very carefully to the question**. Many candidates do not, and achieve only a combination of precious time wasted and an irritated examiner.

Start by examining the system indicated by the examiner in his/her question unless the examiner has stated specifically that you do otherwise. You should be using **all your senses** from the moment you approach the patient. A good doctor is a good **observer**. **Seeing** that there is a sputum pot next to the patient's bed, **hearing** him cough and **smelling** halitosis – all done while the examiner is asking you to examine the chest – should be clues that the patient has bronchiectasis, possibly complicated by anaerobic infection.

Example

"Please examine this patient's chest."

A full respiratory examination with additional relevant signs is sought (i.e. signs of cor pulmonale in emphysema).

Example

*"Please examine the **back** of this patient's chest."*

Do this, but **do not hesitate to go on to look for other signs you may think relevant** afterwards, unless of course you are interrupted. **Always ask yourself why that question was asked in that way**. Be alert to additional signs (a mitral valvotomy scar is often not easily seen from behind the patient, for instance).

You will not be failed for being thorough in your examination but, **if prompted to move on to a specific area, do so quickly**. You have made your point about being thorough and they are trying to save time by guiding you to where the signs are to be found. **Moving on allows you to score more points**. The examiners are not trying to catch you out.

If you have been asked to examine one system, it is quite in order, **having done what you have been asked**, to extend your examination to look for other relevant physical signs. This shows that you understand the significance of your findings and are able to think on your feet, thereby conveying the impression of a knowledgeable and thinking clinician. If you are examining a patient with severe respiratory disease, looking for ankle oedema shows that you know that fluid retention may occur and is of prognostic significance. Similarly in a patient with arthritic hands, looking at the elbows for rheumatoid nodules or patches of psoriasis may help you to diagnose the problem in the hands accurately. Finally in a patient with upper lobe signs on chest examination, a quick look for a Horner's syndrome or wasting of the small muscles of the hand shows that you are alert to a Pancoast tumour.

There are many other situations in which a quick **extension of your examination would be appropriate** in clinical practice. As you practise your Short Cases, ask yourself if there is **anything else that you would normally look for in this situation**?

Answering the question

- Start your answers with the **simple and more common suggestions**, not the rarities. You should explain your findings and what you think they mean and, if possible, arrive at a diagnosis.

- You should also **mention relevant physical signs that you did not find** that you might have expected to find. For example, in a patient with mitral stenosis it is relevant to comment that you did not find any signs of pulmonary hypertension. This shows that you are aware of this complication and that you **understand the implications of your findings**.

- Even if you think you are doing badly, **carry on**. If a particular case has not gone well, try to put it behind you and approach each case as if it is the first that you have seen.

- You are **marked over the full 30 minutes** and can make up lost ground. It is the impression that you make over all the cases that counts, and a good performance in one case will make up for a poor showing in another.

- **It is a popular misconception that you have to get all the diagnoses correct and that a single error will fail you the exam.**

- Examiners are primarily looking for **competence** in clinical examination and a considerate and **thoughtful approach**. If the examiners start asking you difficult questions or pushing you, take heart, you are doing well and they are trying to find out how good you are rather than whether you should just pass the exam.

Never leave the exam or give up part of the way through the examination day. Too many candidates who do this **would have passed**. Challenge your catastrophic predictions and keep going. **Keep your nerve**. At the very least you will gain useful "live" examination practice which will stand you in good stead for any future applications. At best you will pass. Two useful books that allow you to practise a range of Short Cases are *An Aid to the MRCP Short Cases*[1] and *One Hundred Short Cases for the MRCP*.[2]

Key points

- **Keep calm** and always take each Short Case on its own merits. You may think you have done badly but you really don't know, so don't give up – keep going.

- **Listen very carefully to the question.**

- **State the diagnosis** or a differential diagnosis.

- **Give reasons for your diagnosis** with your relevant positive and negative findings on examination.

- **If uncertain as to the diagnosis then give your findings clearly, concisely and honestly** and suggest a differential diagnosis and/or investigations that may help to pinpoint the diagnosis.

- When giving a differential diagnosis try to **list the most likely diagnosis for that patient first**. (systemic lupus erythematosus is more common in young women but is still less common than rheumatoid arthritis. Long-standing itching and jaundice in a woman in her mid-forties is more likely to be primary biliary cirrhosis than metastatic cancer.)

• Be careful with your terminology in front of the patient when referring to cancer or other such emotive subjects such as HIV.

References

[1] R. E. J. Ryder, M. A. Mir and E. A. Freeman, *An Aid to the MRCP Short Cases*, Blackwell Scientific Publications, Oxford, 1996.
[2] K. Gupta,*100 Short Cases for the MRCP*, 2nd edn, Chapman and Hall Medical, London, 1994.

Chapter 11

The viva

Introduction

The viva attempts to make sure that you are clinically safe and sensible, and abreast of current developments in medicine. It offers the examiners a chance to find out both how much you know and, more importantly, to **assess whether you can tackle a problem in a calm and logical manner**, even when the answer is not readily apparent to you.

You will be expected to answer with a level of knowledge that is reasonable for someone of registrar level. Do not be put off if the question is put to you by an examiner who you fear may be a specialist in the area of the question they ask. All that will be expected is for you to have a reasonable overall level of knowledge and to understand the general principles involved. The second examiner is marking your answer, and if he or she considers the question is unreasonable it will be discounted.

Learning for the viva is difficult as a specific task because almost any aspect of medicine may be covered. It is important to keep in mind certain **general principles** to help you with this part of the exam:

> - **Nobody is expected to know everything**. Do not try to bluff your way through this part of the exam; instead try to come over as honest and thoughtful.

Practice is essential to make sure that you communicate what you would do in a variety of clinical situations in a clear and structured way.

- There will be two examiners interviewing you. Both will give you marks and it is important that you should address your remarks to each examiner, not just the one who asked the question. There may be a third person present who would be a trainee MRCP examiner. They will not be involved in the interview itself, and do not contribute to your final mark.

- The examiners are advised to avoid their own specialist chosen subjects. Most (but not all) do this successfully.

Content of the Viva

Just about any medical topic can be asked in the viva, but the questions usually revolve around particular themes:

- **Acute medical problems**, both diagnostic and therapeutic. Know your medical **emergencies**. This should not be a problem as it is closely linked to your job. You have been doing this for years on the wards and in casualty. Say what you would do in practice.

- **Outpatient clinic scenarios**. These are intended to show whether you can collate all available clues and medical knowledge in an effective manner.

- **Basic sciences**. Many examiners are keen on returning to the first principles of physiology, clinical pharmacology and their changes in pathological states. This can include changes specific to the elderly.

- **Clinical pharmacology** (volumes of distribution, etc.) may be disproportionately represented in the viva.

- **Investigation material**. Electrocardiograms (ECGs), and biochemistry results may be the focus of a question. This is less common now as these skills are tested by the written exam.

- **Current themes in the literature**. A number of MRCP examiners believe that the importance of this component is overemphasised by many candidates. Be aware of current trends, however, and be prepared to discuss them with a reasonable level of knowledge.

- You should read through the **editorial leaders in the *British Medical Journal* and the *Lancet*** for the last 18 months and/or *Archives of Disease in Childhood* if you are sitting the Paediatrics exam. This can help highlight current changes in clinical practice and "hot" topics in the organisation and structure of the National Health Service (NHS). You do not need to read every article in great detail but it will help you to be aware of what is topical. It may also be helpful to read the medical sections in the Sunday newspapers as these often deal with new advances and controversies and are a quick way of keeping abreast of what is going on.

- **Medical ethics** or politics.

- **Your opinions** regarding current affairs related to the NHS. Your opinion may be different to that held by the examiner and it is best to give the pros and cons to both sides of the argument. Use a balanced argument.

- Be prepared to answer an open question (example: "*What do you think is the most important clinical development in the past 10 years?*"). Prepare for this type of question. It is worth the trouble and can change a nightmare question into a joy.

- **Do not argue**. You can give your answer and your reasons for that answer, but do not antagonise the examiners.

Allocation of marks in the viva

The two examiners are asked to examine on four separate topics in both the Adult and Paediatric exams using both sections below.

Adult and Paediatric exam viva

Section A
(Two topics are chosen from:)

1. Management of emergencies.
2. Diagnostic problem.
3. Planning management of chronic disease.
4. Recent literature including developments.

Section B
(Two topics are covered from:)

1. Physiology and physiopathology.
2. Communication with patients and relatives, ethical issues.
3. Psychology, social and behavioural.
4. Clinical research or audit/resource management/statistics.

Examiners initially mark each candidate individually, and then agree on a final joint mark.

Viva Techniques

The examiners have questions prepared for the viva. They are, however, dependent on the candidate for the follow-up questions. If you list a rare cause of a particular symptom, be prepared to be asked about it. In trying to convey all the information that you know it is easy not to think this far ahead. This can be improved with practice. Answering in the viva is a little like answering questions in court. **Think where every response may lead and beware**.

- Learn to **structure your answer** so that you present information clearly and concisely.

- Learn to realise and **communicate what you know**.

- Try to direct the questions towards your **stronger areas** of proficiency.

A number of techniques are central to answering effectively:

- It is essential to be **systematic and organised** in your approach to answering in the viva.

- **Do not restrict** your answers so that you answer only one part of the question. It is easy to make the mistake of answering on only one area or aspect of the problem, thus going down a "blind alley" and running out of things to say. **Keep your thinking broad and at a basic level initially**.

- **Do not say too much**. You may talk yourself into trouble. Never open a door that you are not prepared to walk through.

- Try to avoid a lengthy pause. Try to **keep your answers simple to start with** and then build on this foundation with additional knowledge.

You can **gain thinking time** by saying what the main thrust of the question involves (thinking out loud). Comment on:

1. **Issues**: What are the main issues raised by the question?

•   Diagnosis, management and investigation.

•   Patient issues (compliance, etc.).

2. **Information**: Do you need any more information? Where from?

•   To make the diagnosis.

•   To decide on treatment. What are the benefits and risks of treatment?

•   Impact on the patient.

•   Impact on other people (e.g. carers, etc.).

*"This question involves a number of different **issues**. It raises the importance of being sure of the original diagnosis, the need for a full assessment, and also the difficulties of treating those with chronic chest disease . . . "*

*"In this case I would wish to gather further **information** in order to clarify the diagnosis. I would arrange the following diagnostic tests . . . "*

This has the advantage of showing the examiners that you can pick out the **key points** quickly and have a firm grasp of the essentials of care.

Another way of helping you gain valuable thinking time is **to talk yourself into the situation** and allow the examiners to realise that you grasp the key features of the case:

"If I was asked to go and see this case in casualty, I would start thinking about how to manage the case on the way there . . . "

Example

What are the causes of a big spleen?

It is impossible to answer this question well without **structuring your response**. The candidate who begins to reel off an infinite list of possible causes, starting with the most obscure, will exasperate the examiners. You do not wish to do this.

Qualities of a "bad" answer

- The answer **lacks structure and is presented badly** with comments such as *"I meant to say . . . oh yes, and also"*, etc.

- Eye contact with the examiner is avoided by **staring at the floor** when the answer is not known.

- The candidate clearly **lacks confidence** and comes over as someone who cannot make a decision or show effective clinical judgement. He or she has no answer to follow-up questions which seem to floor them.

- A list of responses is given that **takes no account of the relative frequency and importance** of the conditions.

- There is no **definite end-point** to the answer, which rambles on ineffectively.

- A major cause is completely left out.

- If increasingly rare causes are all given towards the end of the answer, this invites follow-up questions about the things you know least.

- Never say *"There are ten causes of a big spleen"*. It will not come over well if you can remember only six.

Qualities of a "good" answer

- Impose an effective structure to the answer.

- Make eye contact with the examiners in a non-challenging way.

- Provide a list of responses that covers all the important and common conditions.

- Make sure there is a clear end-point to the answer.

- Speak clearly and confidently, showing a professional manner.

Example

"Several disease processes can cause an enlarged spleen, for example:"

- **Infective** causes such as malaria, glandular fever, etc.

- **Storage disorders** such as . . .

- **Malignancies** such as . . .

- **Cardiovascular** problems such as . . .

- **Haematological** causes such as . . .

- **Portal hypertension** secondary to . . .

- Demonstrate **confidence** and an organised mind.

- Gain thinking time by using this structured approach.

- The clear structure means that the examiners will not insist on an exhaustive list.

- Knowing where you are heading in your presentation adds to your confidence and reduces panic.

- Answering in a structured way excuses you from having to rank your answers in order of frequency or importance. You can always add comments such as *"I think that malaria is the most likely cause in this case because of . . . "* to clarify this.

- Interesting information can be held back to satisfy follow-up questions.

- Friendly follow-up questions can be encouraged by giving less obtrusive causes towards the end of the answer.

- The answer comes to a **natural end**.

- It doesn't really matter if you miss a category.

Example

"What do you know about neurofibromatosis?"

- Neurofibromatosis is an uncommon, autosomal dominant, inherited, condition.

- It exists in two major forms, types 1 and 2.

- Patients often present with dermatological features, which are . . .

- Complications include . . .

Many candidates faced with a question about a topic with which they are unfamiliar panic and go to pieces. They often actually know all that is required of them and yet think they should know more. Structuring your answer will allow limited information to be presented in a meaningful manner. Regular practice at answering questions will significantly improve your ability to structure and present answers.

Reducing anxiety

- When candidates are nervous they tend to talk too fast. This substantially reduces thinking time and suggests a lack of confidence.

- Anxiety makes structuring answers difficult, and you may overwhelm the examiner with information. This may lead to confusion and errors in the answer and irritate your examiners.

- When asked a question, purposefully **take a few seconds to think** about the answer. Try to talk slowly; pause between each sentence of your answer.

- **Answer with confidence**. If the candidate appears under-confident or unsure then the examiner is also less convinced that he or she knows the subject. Certainty comes with practice and knowledge. **You can still be confident even if you don't know the answer to a question**. Say **where** you would go for the information or who you would discuss the case with for further clarification. For example, if you do not know what drugs you can safely prescribe in pregnancy, you can say this. It is quite reasonable to say *"I would contact the pharmacy and Drug Information and ask for further information"*. At times it would be very appropriate to discuss a clinical problem with your boss or seek a specialist opinion. If so, say so.

- Confidence is very important but **over-confidence is potentially disastrous**. A candidate who is over-confident and who tries to bluff their way through a subject they know little about is potentially dangerous in the clinical situation. **You are more likely to worry the examiners if you give the**

impression that you believe you can treat every-thing *all* of the time.

- If you find the questions getting more difficult, do not be disheartened. The examiners see a lot of candidates and will enjoy one who actually does well. They may, therefore, ask increasingly difficult questions to determine how good the candidate is. Thus in this part of the exam, if the examiners seem to be building up the pressure it is because the examinee is doing well, not because they are doing badly. **Do not get the wrong impression.** Candidates always think the worst, but should not panic.

- In the viva, the examiners may well ask a question to which he does not expect the candidate to know the answer. The purpose of this is to determine how the candidate thinks and how they would approach the unknown. The exam is not designed only to test the recall of factual information, but also to ensure that the candidate knows how to approach a patient, knows how to think through a problem, how to deal with the unexpected, and in essence, how to be a good clinician.

- As a MRCP candidate **you are not expected to know everything**. If you do not know the answer, admit that you do not, but try not to do it too often.

- **If the examiners appear to disagree with you strongly**, be prepared to consider other possibilities. Be willing to discuss other diagnostic or treatment options. **Never get into an argument**, but if you consider that you are correct, you should review with the examiners the reasons for and against each of the possibilities, and the reasons why you wish for the time being to stick to your first decision. Always show that if more information became available, or the person changed, that you would be willing to reconsider. **Never let yourself become angry or confrontational with an examiner**. If you do this, you will fail.

The principles of answering questions effectively in the viva are illustrated by the following example:

Example

"How would you investigate a 40-year-old man with hypertension?"

Although you should be able to give a full and extensive answer, as soon as it is apparent that you are knowledgeable in this area the examiners are likely to guide you with leading questions which can produce more of a "tennis match" in place of a monologue. The following illustrates one possible answer to this question. It is unlikely that you will be able to give the full answer. The examiners are likely to interrupt and guide you into specific areas. This is normal, but can be disconcerting. You should try to lead the questioning into areas about which you are knowledgeable and comfortable. If you don't know a definition of hypertension then try to focus on the clinical aspects about which you are familiar.

Possible answer

- First, you must examine the question and **define hypertension**, both for the examiners and yourself. This will clarify the management for yourself.

- Your **immediate action** would depend upon the degree of hypertension. Hypertension can be grouped into mild (> 90 mmHg diastolic), moderate (> 100 mgHg diastolic) and severe (>110 mmHg diastolic). The World Health Organisation suggests a level of 160/95 as the upper limit of normal, but a diastolic level of 100 mmHg (phase V) was used by the British Hypertension Society Working Party 1989, with treatment at this level having been shown as beneficial.

- Comment that his relatively young age makes you suspicious of a **secondary cause for the hypertension** rather than the diagnosis being benign essential hypertension.

- **Start your assessment** with a full history looking for risk factors, including family history (for hypertension, ischaemic heart disease, stroke, hypercholesterolaemia and renal disease), smoking, diabetes, ischaemic heart disease and peripheral vascular disease. Palpitations and postural hypotension occur in phaeochromocytomas.

- A **thorough examination**, including recording the blood pressure in all limbs on your first appointment, looking for discrepancies. Look specifically for radio-radial or radiofemoral delay. Aortic or machinery murmurs can also be found in coarctation of the aorta. Femoral pulses may be impalpable. Look for polycystic kidneys. Cushing's syndrome has characteristic features on examination.

- You will need to **repeat recordings** of the blood pressure over an interval of several months before commencing therapy, unless the recordings are very high.

- In addition, your response depends on the presence of **end-organ damage** at presentation. Fundoscopy for retinopathy and urine dipstick testing for haematoproteinuria will alert you to the **need for earlier intervention**.

- Then you can move on to **simple investigations** including biochemistry for renal impairment and diabetes, lipid profile for assessment of risk factors, and electrocardiography for left ventricular hypertrophy.

- **Further investigation** would probably be limited to patients who you suspect as having a secondary cause: i.e. 24-hour urine collections to investigate the possibility of Cushing's syndrome or a phaeochromocytoma, and estimation of lying and ambulant renin and aldosterone levels for Conn's syndrome. Renal ultrasonography will show up polycystic kidneys or unequally sized kidneys in established renovascular disease. An intravenous pyelogram, a renal perfusion scan, renal arteriogram, adrenal computed tomogram or renal biopsy may be necessary according to earlier investigations.

Mock Vivas

It is important to practise **doing mock vivas**. Many candidates find them surprisingly difficult, simply because they have not become familiar with the technique. In fact they are very simple, because all you have to say is what **you** would do in practice. You have been solving similar problems whilst "on call" and on the wards for the last few years. Be sensible and safe, and you will pass.

A source of questions that may be useful for practice is *An Aid to the MRCP Viva*.[1]

Usually candidates' nerves are worst while waiting for the exam: you may well find that you feel a lot better once the exam is underway. Using these techniques and making sure that you have practised this style of examination before the actual day will also boost your confidence and settle your nerves.

Key points

- Be aware of the range of possible questions.

- Be clinically sensible and safe.

- Say what you would do in practice.

- Be divergent in your thinking and avoid going down a blind alley.

- Organise your answer clearly.

- Gain thinking time by considering what further **information** you require and what the key **issues** involved in the case are. **Talking yourself "into" the clinical scenario** may also help.

- Do not be dogmatic.

- Where appropriate, say that you would seek advice or information from others with more experience in that area.

Reference

[1] M. A. Mir, E. A. Freeman and R. E. J. Ryder, *An Aid to the MRCP Viva,* Churchill Livingstone, London, 1992.

Part IV

The Paediatric exam

Chapter 12

The clinical exam in Paediatrics

Introduction

If you wish to pursue a career in some aspect of Paediatrics it will be necessary for you to sit, and pass, the Membership exams of the Royal College of Physicians. Indeed, once the Calman proposals are implemented, it will be necessary to pass the MRCP exams in order to become a specialist registrar in Paediatrics.

Paediatricians must sit both Parts I and II of the MRCP. Those who wish to be paediatricians will apply for and sit either the identical Part I exam as everyone else or the Paediatrics Part I. The techniques and approach necessary to pass this part of the exam are outlined in **Chapter 3**.

In the MRCP Part II exams, potential paediatricians sit a paper containing paediatric topics. Those who are planning a career in adult medicine or a related specialty sit the Adult exam. There are some questions, usually concerning adolescent patients, which appear in both papers. It is not necessary for paediatricians to sit the Paediatric exam, or indeed for Adult physicians to sit the Adult exam – both have equal status.

Much of what has been written for the Adult clinical exam in Part III of this book is also true for the Paediatrics exam. We suggest that you read that section of the book several times in addition to this chapter. Useful books covering the written exams include

Grey cases for Paediatric Examinations[1], Data interpretation for Paediatric Examinations[2], and 100 Paediatric Picture tests.[3]

General Paediatric Clinical Techniques

The Paediatric exam is very similar to the Adult exam, although there are several important differences of which you need to be aware.

- Be opportunistic. It is more important to be **child friendly** than to stick to a rigid examination protocol.

- Remember young children often need to **gain your trust** before they will let you examine them – a few moments spent talking to them is often very effective.

- Try to avoid asking permission from young children: if they say "no" you are in trouble; ask the parent.

- **Warm your hands** before examining babies.

- Under no circumstances cause **pain**.

- Try to **avoid talking about frightening subjects in front of children**: children listen well and have vivid imaginations.

- **Don't trust children**. For example, if you are testing vision make sure one eye is properly covered.

- The exam venue should have all the equipment you require for your examination; take your stethoscope, but not a suitcase full of toys. It may be helpful to take an auroscope and ophthalmoscope with which you are comfortable.

- Be able to examine the child confidently and efficiently.

- Talk to the child and try to establish a relationship with them if they are old enough.

- Don't be afraid to talk to the child and parent.

- Be 100% prepared to be asked to do a **developmental examination**. Practise in front of colleagues until you are happy with your technique.

- Know what to do if the child cries or refuses to co-operate.

- Never examine a child's genitals unless you are specifically asked to do so.

- Urine dipstick testing and microscopy should be a routine part of your clinical examination.

- Always act professionally.

Some aspects of Paediatrics, particularly child protection work, requires a senior opinion as part of the routine assessment. Asking for this is an appropriate request in these circumstances.

The Short Cases

- Listen to the examiners' questions very carefully and answer succinctly and directly.

- Time spent **inspecting** is probably the most productive time and the most neglected. This can buy you enough time to organise your thoughts.

- The more cases you see the better. You have more chances to score points.

- Do not artificially make your physical findings fit your presumed diagnosis. In real life, cases may present a mixed picture. It is quite reasonable to say this in the exam.

- If you are unsure of the diagnosis, present the positive and the important negative findings.

- If you don't know the answer to a question, say so. Do not waffle. Time is very important: do not waste any.

- Practise, practise, practise.

Spotting subjects

In the Paediatrics exam, you are most likely to see a variety of different cases. Some areas are either seen commonly in clinical practice, or represent areas that are viewed as being of greater clinical importance. Many of the clinical cases will have been to the exam many times before. Prepare yourself well for the more common cases. These include:

- Cystic fibrosis.

- Failure to thrive.

- Infant asthma, etc.

System spot

Make sure you are competent at examination skills. Pre-prepare system examinations so that you can carry these out effectively and efficiently.

Examples

"Examine this child for a squint."
"Examine this child's seventh facial nerve."

"Examine this child's legs, etc."

Bear in mind basic examination techniques:

- Be polite to the patient and the examiners.

- Avoid the temptation to argue with or correct the examiners.

- Try not to listen to what is happening around you. Other candidates may be wrong in their conclusions.

- The exam is often a shock for first-time candidates; it may appear chaotic. Try not to be distracted.

- You may be rushed, interrupted and not allowed to get into a rhythm. Be prepared for this; if you are asked for a diagnosis give one, and not all of your findings.

- The Short Cases should not be approached with only survival in mind. This is your opportunity to display your knowledge and clinical acumen – don't waste it.

THE LONG CASE

The best practice for the Long Case is to see children/patients in the outpatient department and present them to senior colleagues. Practise presenting long cases to other exam candidates.

Have a pre-prepared structure to your presentation that examiners will recognise. One possible structure is suggested below:

- Presenting complaint.

- History of presenting complaint.

- Review of systems.

- Past medical history.

- Drugs/allergies.

- Family history.

- Social history.

- Physical examination (key positive and important negative findings that are of diagnostic importance).

Do not forget important basic information, e.g. **birth history, allergies and immunisation record**.

- Senior house officers particularly and junior doctors in general, deal mainly with acute problems; remember that the exam is more likely to be about chronic problems.

- Many Long Cases have appeared in the exam before; if you have time, ask the parent if there is **anything you have forgotten to ask** or which they think is important that you don't know.

Allow yourself 10–15 minutes towards the end of the Long Case to **structure** your thoughts and presentation. Formulate a management plan, including differential diagnosis, investigations, management and prognosis as outlined in **Chapter 9**. Pay particular attention to areas that are stressed in Paediatrics.

Example

"What investigations would you wish to carry out on this child?"

These could include an assessment of the following areas:

- Physical.

- Psychological and developmental (e.g. IQ test, psychological reports).

- Social: Social work reports of the home circumstances, risk of physical, sexual or other abuse or neglect; school reports, etc.

You are most likely to get a child with a **chronic illness** as a Long Case. Remember that the management of chronic illness involves a lot more than medication. Be very familiar with all other forms of support and treatment. Always consider a three-systems approach to management:

1. **Physical treatments**: medication, operations, antibiotics, etc.

2. **Psychological**: Specific referral to a child psychologist or psychiatrist may sometimes be indicated. Occupational therapists or physiotherapists may be helpful in some cases (for example, to improve motor skills and co-ordination, or to treat cystic fibrosis).

3. **Social**: Information about the illness and support for the child and family are always necessary in both short-term and more chronic conditions.

A useful way of understanding the problems a child with a chronic illness may have is to ask the parent to describe in detail a **typical day**, and the **effects** of the illness on the child and family. Useful questions may include:

- What have they/you been forced to stop as a result of their illness?

- What would they/you be able to do if they were no longer ill?

When you are being examined, always be totally truthful to the examiners. If you are asked a specific question that you do not know the answer to, say so. If you have forgotten to examine the spine or eyes, say so. **Never make up an answer** as you will be discovered. Instead, apologise for not having the answer; say why you should have asked the question, and say that on this one occasion you have forgotten.

If you do not know what the diagnosis is in the Long Case, don't panic – **nobody** may know the diagnosis. It is important to know how to establish a diagnosis and to be able to manage a patient without a diagnosis.

A useful book is Clinical Paediatrics for Postgraduate Examinations.[4]

The Viva

The viva is the most difficult part of the clinical exam because it is the most different from normal day-to-day experience. It is quite unusual for junior doctors to be asked direct factual questions, so it is not surprising that their skills at answering such questions are generally poor. The only way to improve these skills is to practise answering as many viva questions as possible. A useful book is the Paediatric MRCP Viva.[5] Time spent in practice vivas is not only appropriate for the viva but also for the other parts of the clinical exam. You should also read **Chapter 11** to improve your technique.

Key points

- Practice is essential. Practise, practise, practise.
- A good basic knowledge and understanding is all you need to pass the exam.
- Subject spot.
- Try to identify your weak areas.
- Learn to structure answers clearly.
- Learn to answer with confidence. Communicate clearly and act professionally.
- Do not underestimate yourself.
- Remember this is your opportunity to show the examiners that you are an effective clinician.

References

1 D. J. Field, J. Stroobant, A. Fenton, I. Maconchie and C. O'Calloghan, *Grey cases for Paediatric Examinations*, Churchill Livingstone, London, 1995.
2 C. O'Callaghan and T. Stephenson, *Data interpretation for Paediatric Examinations*, Churchill Livingstone, London, 1994.
3 A. P. Winnow, M. Gatzoulis and G. Supramanian, *100 Paediatric Picture tests*, Churchill Livingstone, London, 1994.
4 T. Stephenson and H. Wallace, *Clinical Paediatrics for Postgraduate Examinations*, 2nd edn, Churchill Livingstone, London, 1995.
5 A. Cade, A. Shetty and T. S. Tinklin, *Paediatric MRCP Viva*, Churchill Livingstone, London, 1995.

Appendix 1

What if you fail?
Trying again

Siân McIver

"You may be disappointed if you fail, but you are doomed if you don't try."

(Beverley Sills, b. 1929, American opera singer and
manager)

After you have taken the exam, the results will come out a number of weeks after the multiple choice question paper for Part I or quite soon after the viva for Part II. Even if you think the exam went badly, during these few weeks you may have convinced your friends and family that you **know** you have failed and are resolved to retake it at the next sitting, but you will not have convinced yourself of this. Up until that last minute before the "fat envelope" hits the hall carpet, there will still be the glimmer of hope that you have passed.

Unfortunately, the truth is that more people will fail each part of the exam than will pass. There will be those who have laboured long and hard covering even the most obscure parts of huge tomes in great detail who will have to go through this dispiriting experience. It is at this point that the most negative and unrealistic thoughts may emerge:

- *"I'll never pass." "What happens if I do this on my next three attempts? I'll be barred for life."*

- *"My wife will leave me if I have to put her through that again and I'll never see my children again!"*

Such thoughts are both **unhelpful and inaccurate,** but are part of the normal adjustment reaction that will take place. At this point, if you have just failed Part II, reading the feedback can help to challenge these beliefs. You will find that **you do have some strengths** and it will be necessary to remind yourself of this.

Ask senior colleagues if they have any thoughts as to why you failed. Encourage them to be honest.

Letting other people know the results can be one of the most difficult undertakings, as this may well be the first important exam you have failed. It is worth taking some time telling the people you care about so that they can appreciate what a blow this has been to you and may offer you support. At work, try to remember that probably about half of the consultants that you work with will also have had to resit this exam themselves, yet you could probably not tell which ones they were. Colleagues may try to ascertain whether you have passed or not by studying you intensely from a distance before deciding whether to ask you. Some may be sympathetic and supportive; for others, try to learn a short but positive reply.

Failing a postgraduate exam is a **major life event** and you will be more likely to succeed at a resit attempt if you allow yourself to recover emotionally first. **Be kind to yourself, get plenty of sleep and spend some time doing your favourite things**. At a practical level there may be things that you have postponed due to the exam which, if you don't attend to now, may get in the way of your revision. You may need to have central heating fitted or to see some long-neglected relatives. Now is also the time to sort out your finances. Resits are expensive: make sure you claim for all the expenses you were entitled to from your first attempt, and remember that some Trusts will pay for revision courses for resit candidates. This is also a good time to get your CV up to date – you may end up applying for a job near the time of your resit and you won't welcome the diversion of sorting it out then. Keep a copy on disk so that when you pass the exam, you can simply fill in the date. Not only will these things ease the burden on your time nearer the resit, they will also help to restore some **perspective** to your life. The exam – even your career – is only one part of life but it is possible to become totally immersed in it and lose sight of other more important things.

Whenever plans go awry it is important to try to find out **why it happened**. You must evaluate the situation because, if you don't know why things went wrong the first time, it is possible that you may make the same mistakes again. You must be honest with yourself when answering the question "Why did I fail?". Most people who fail know exactly why they failed - learn from your experience. Could it be that you had not looked carefully enough at central areas and concentrated on peripheral subjects, or did you skimp on books and courses? Another possibility is that you did not book your study leave early enough and, not only did you end up without any time off to revise before the exam, but you were working harder than usual, covering for your more organised colleagues who had booked theirs well in advance.

Even those who know the facts of the subjects inside out may fail as a **result of poor exam technique**. If this is not the cause of your failure then you may have to consider the possibility that your failure was caused by the simple error of just not working hard enough. In other words, you can plan, organise, timetable and buy books until it becomes an art form – but you do need to leave time to study as well. Beware of focusing all your efforts on the part of the exam that you failed. It would be very upsetting to pass this with flying colours only to fail on another part at the next attempt. The Royal Colleges run a scheme which offers exam counselling to some candidates who have failed. This is generally helpful and it is advisable to pursue this if it is offered.

To move on from here you will need to **motivate yourself** and decide that this is really the direction that you want to go in. It may be that you were sitting the exam for the **wrong reasons** or that you were actually sitting the **wrong exam**, and now may be a good time to review this. If you do decide to alter your career direction at this time, make sure that you are making this decision for **positive reasons, rather than as an avoidance strategy**. Even if you are sure that you are doing the right exam, it may not be the best **time** for you to resit it – for instance, if you are just about to have a new addition to the family. However, generally speaking it is probably best to pay for the resit while the information from the last attempt is still fresh in your mind.

Once you have decided to attempt the exam again, dedication is required and a revision timetable may help. Not only will it ensure that you cover each topic but it will also mean that you can timetable breaks where you are free from the guilt of not working. Some people find that meeting with other people who are sitting the exam to form a study group can help: sitting with a large pot of coffee and some chocolate biscuits can really help the information to go in. Check out which study courses are available to you and apply for this and private study leave as soon as possible. Consider attending a specific Examination Techniques course if you feel that the problem is an inability to communicate what you know effectively.

In conclusion, if you fail the exam try to:

- **Evaluate** the reasons why you failed.

- **Motivate** yourself to press on and do the resit.

- **Dedicate** yourself to the hard work of revision.

- **Appreciate** the importance of exam techniques so that you present what you know to its best effect.

"If you have made mistakes . . . there is always another chance for you . . . you may have a fresh start any moment you choose, for this thing we call "failure" is not the falling down but the staying down."

(Mary Pickford (1893–1979), American actress)

Appendix 2

What are Mind Maps and how can they help with the exam?

Kevin Appleton

You will be already aware of your strengths and weaknesses when it comes to learning for exams. You will probably use techniques which you have (successfully) used over the years. Successful techniques allow you to structure, organise and integrate new information with the information that you already know in order to make learning meaningful. This is important because, particularly with the Part II exam, it is a practical impossibility to read through everything again in the few days before the exam. It is important to focus on key facts, so that these may be concentrated on, in order to reduce the amount of reading you have to do when the work is revised.

Common and effective techniques to help you reduce the quantity of information you have to learn include writing short summary notes or using highlighter pens to focus in on key facts. Another less common approach is Mind Mapping. This is not an approach that everyone will find intuitively appealing; however, some people find this approach to be a very helpful way of organising and learning information.

Mind Maps® are colourful, branching pictures or diagrams that can help your memory, thinking and organisation of ideas and information. They can make study more efficient by condensing more facts on to a single sheet so that very large amounts of information may be revised very quickly. In Mind Map® 1 the assessment and treatment of alcohol addiction is covered, together with the ways that alcohol problems can lead to presentation to the medical services. To maximise the effectiveness of Mind Maps® it is necessary to produce your own so that each subheading of the Mind Map® will trigger off associated pieces of information in your own memory. If you had Mind Map® 1 in the Short Cases or Viva, you would be able to answer most questions on this topic.

Mind Maps® work by increasing the cross-connections and associations of stored information in memory. They use images or key words to anchor information and to trigger associations. It is possible to hold entire Mind Maps® in visual memory by this method – and they are fun to use, making learning more enjoyable and revision less tedious. By using different modes of memory storage (e.g. factual, visual and colour), they increase the modalities and ways in which information can be remembered, whereas linear text uses only one such modality.

How to Create your own Mind Maps

It is better to draw Mind Maps® across the horizontal axis of the page, as the structure spreads out better this way. Start with a central image or icon. Recalling this from visual memory will trigger your recall of the whole map. Next, arrange main headings or key words around this from the centre of the page. Subheadings, lists and further details can then be added to each branch.

One heading or icon (e.g. trauma as in Mind Map® 1) will come to represent, in your own mind, many other additional responses (subdural, penetrating, etc.). These act as anchors for surrounding text and help you to recall this additional information efficiently. Well-organised information should result in an aesthetically pleasing map whereas poorly organised information will look a mess and will be less well recalled. To structure the content clearly on paper means that it must also be structured clearly in your mind, so that drawing out the diagram is itself an effective means of revision. This is illustrated by Mind Map® 2, which summarises the use and production of Mind Maps.® You will see that the key

Mind Map® 1. Alcohol: assessment, complications and treatment

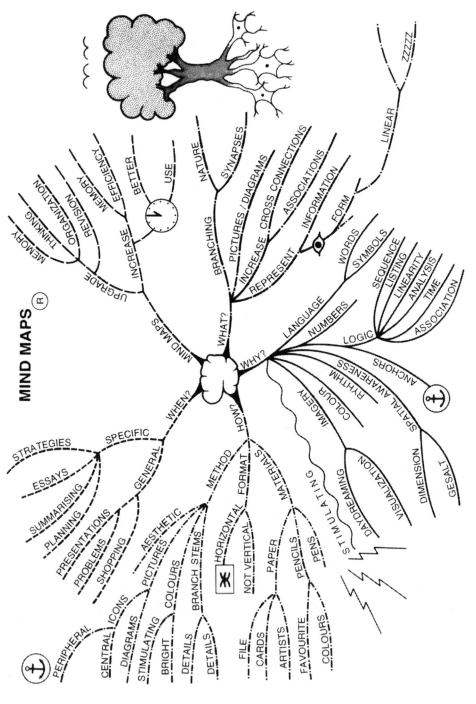

Mind Map® **2**. Mind maps summarised

elements of the linear text you are now reading are clearly and concisely summarised on one sheet of paper. This is both information rich and very quickly read. If this is the case for this section of the book, could it also be the case for your exam revision?

Because Mind Maps® can be used to summarise large amounts of information into a manageable form, this information can be reviewed very quickly just before the exam, maximising the recency effect. It is therefore possible to revise the content of even large books in only a short period of time.

A full account of the use of Mind Maps® can be found in *The Mind Map Book.*[1]

References

[1] T Busan and B Busan *The Mind Map Book. Busan*, BBC Books, London, 1993.
[R] ®Mind Map is the Registered Trade Mark of the Buzan Organisation.

Index